INVASION OF THE PROSTATE SNATCHERS

INVASION
OF THE
PROSTATE
SNATCHERS

NO MORE
UNNECESSARY BIOPSIES,
RADICAL TREATMENT OR LOSS
OF SEXUAL POTENCY

RALPH H. BLUM
MARK SCHOLZ, MD

OTHER PRESS

NEW YORK

Copyright © 2010 Ralph H. Blum and Mark Scholz

Production Editor: *Yvonne E. Cárdenas*

Book design: *Simon M. Sullivan*

This book was set in 10.5 pt Electra by Alpha Design & Composition
of Pittsfield, NH.

10 9 8 7 6 5 4 3 2

LIBRARY OF CONGRESS CATALOGING-IN-PUBLICATION DATA
Blum, Ralph, 1932–
Invasion of the prostate snatchers : no more unnecessary biopsies, radical treatment
or loss of sexual potency / Ralph H. Blum, Mark Scholz.
p. ; cm.
Includes bibliographical references and index.
ISBN 978-1-59051-342-2 (hardcover) — ISBN 978-1-59051-385-9 (e-book)
1. Prostate—Cancer—Popular works.   2. Prostate—Cancer—Surgery—
Popular works.   I. Scholz, Mark.   II. Title.
[DNLM: 1. Prostatic Neoplasms—therapy—Personal Narratives.   2. Early
Detection of Cancer—Personal Narratives.   3. Erectile Dysfunction—
prevention & control—Personal Narratives.   4. Prostatic Neoplasms—
diagnosis—Personal Narratives.   5. Unnecessary Procedures—adverse
effects—Personal Narratives. WJ 762 B658i 2010]
RC280.P7358 2010
616.99'463—dc22   2010005194

DISCLAIMER

The views expressed by the authors of this book are not intended as a substitute for
medical advice, diagnosis or treatment provided by the reader's personal physicians
about any matters regarding prostate cancer. The authors and the publisher
specifically disclaim any liability for any loss or risk that is incurred as a consequence
of the use and application of any of the contents of this book.

Although the stories in this book are true, certain names and occupations of
individuals mentioned in the book have been changed to protect their privacy.

The authors have made every effort to provide accurate telephone numbers
and Internet addresses at the time of publication, but neither the publisher nor
the authors assume any responsibility for errors, or for changes that occur after
publication of this book. Moreover, the publisher does not have any control
over and does not assume any responsibility for author or third-party Web sites
or their content.

Although the book contains a listing entitled "Prostate Oncologists," inclusion
of these oncologists should not be interpreted as their endorsing the views
expressed in this book.

CONTENTS

While writing this book, I have become ever more aware of the vital role played by women in men's healing, and the support of all the loving partners whose lives have been impacted by this disease. May our work help to sustain and encourage you.

—RALPH BLUM

I want to dedicate this book to the nearly two hundred thousand men diagnosed with prostate cancer each year. And especially to all my patients over these past sixteen years.

—MARK SCHOLZ

INVASION OF THE PROSTATE SNATCHERS

PROLOGUE

RALPH BLUM

> As for the prostate gland itself? It's like Bulgaria. No one is quite sure just where it is or what goes on there.
>
> — HAL ACKERMAN, *My Generation Magazine*

For over twenty years, I have lived with prostate cancer. During that time, the most important thing I learned is that I was blessed with the form of the disease that was "Low Risk" rather than "Aggressive," a cancer that is slow growing and almost never fatal. Which is why I fully expect to depart this earth a jolly old man, in my sleep, after a lovely day in the country with my honey and a few cherished friends.

My long and often humbling affiliation with prostate cancer began in Malibu, California, on a summer afternoon in 1990, when my family doctor, Jeff Harris, pulled on his latex glove, gave me his slow, surfer's smile, and suggested that I "drop 'em and assume the position." It was part of my regular checkup, the annual uncomfortable but necessary experience of the DRE or Digital Rectal Exam, the old doctor-inserts-finger-up-your-butt ritual most men over the age of forty-five are familiar with.

I was fifty-eight. I'd probably had half a dozen normal DREs. Then on that sunny afternoon, while giving my prostate a conscientious probing, Jeff found a lump. And because my PSA was slightly elevated for my age, he wanted me to have a biopsy. Since without a biopsy you would not know for sure if there was cancer, I grudgingly agreed.

Jeff referred me to a Los Angeles urologist — who I will call Dr. Danforth — to do a needle biopsy of the lump. Lying there on the surgeon's table, I was sweating. My attitude was already surly and mistrustful. I was having a primitive reaction to letting some stranger cut out fragments, cores of my flesh. Here's this guy I've known for only twenty minutes going at it with his transistorized jackhammer: Core! . . . Core! . . . And he's hurting me, and I'm lying there rigid, thinking: *What if we're really pissing off those*

1

cancer cells? Core! . . . Core! *What if the shock triggers the diseased little mothers into making a run for it—to get as far way from this demolition site as they can?* Core! . . . Core! . . . *What are the chances that if there is cancer, he's actually spreading it!*

Three days later, Jeff called with the results of some blood tests. Then he announced almost casually, "By the way, Dr. Danforth wants to redo the biopsy."

"You've got to be kidding!"

"Afraid I'm serious."

"Whoa! Redo it! Why?"

Short pause. "Seems he got crush artifact."

"What is that supposed to mean?"

"The specimens he removed were crushed."

"Crushed? You mean he blew it?"

"Something like that."

After I hung up, I just sat there. *Redo the biopsy! Redo the bloody biopsy! Fat chance!* I took a long, cold shower. Then I rang Dr. Danforth's office. They asked when I wanted to reschedule. I felt like suggesting that they assemble the cores already in their possession, wrap them in their bill, have the doctor assume the position, then insert the whole thing.

Instead, I said I'd be in touch.

As with most things, there was a good side to all this. Regardless of the lump and my slightly elevated PSA, and despite the urologist's report evaluating the lump as "suspicious for well-differentiated adenocarcinoma" and his recommending surgery—even *without* another biopsy—thanks to that crush artifact there was no "proof positive." No way to be absolutely certain that I had prostate cancer. My gut feeling was: *Time is on my side!* So I decided there was no point worrying.

It was nine years before I submitted to another biopsy.

INTRODUCTION

MARK SCHOLZ, MD

> My father used to say to me, "Whenever you get into a jam, whenever you get into a crisis or an emergency . . . become the calmest person in the room and you'll be able to figure your way out of it."
>
> —RUDOLPH GIULIANI

"I'm scheduled for surgery next week, but my doctor says the operation can make me impotent—and the cancer may come back anyway. I really don't like the odds."

Every year, nearly a half-million men in the United States and Europe are diagnosed with prostate cancer. Most of them are under the terrifying impression that they are about to die. They don't realize that prostate cancer is different from other cancers. In reality, only about one out of seven men with the disease—perhaps 15%—are truly at risk. New research shows that there is an indolent variety of the disease that is not life threatening, a type that can be safely monitored without immediate treatment.

My days consist of providing counsel to desperate men seeking an alternative to a treatment that can deprive them of normal urinary and sexual function. When a man is diagnosed with prostate cancer, he is immediately confronted with conflicting opinions, partial information and doctors with a penchant for surgery. There was a time, now past, when surgery was considered an appropriate remedy. In fact, surgery was termed the "gold standard" of treatments. Thank God, we are off that gold standard.

The tragedy is that most men don't know this.

Research has now proven that many men who were "cured" by surgery had a form of the disease that was never destined to threaten their lives. Out of 50,000 radical prostatectomies performed every year in the United States alone, *more than 40,000 are unnecessary*. In other words, the vast majority of men with prostate cancer would have lived just as long without any operation at all. Most did not need to have their sexuality cut out.

3

Why, then, are so many prostate operations still being performed? The answer to this question is rarely discussed but easy to comprehend. Urologists, who are surgeons, dominate the field of prostate cancer. This is the *only* type of cancer where this is the case. Medical oncologists, the cancer specialists who manage all the other types of cancers, such as breast, colon and lung, are almost never involved in the management of newly diagnosed prostate cancer. Therefore I am something of an anomaly, a medical oncologist totally devoted to treating men with prostate cancer. There are over 10,000 medical oncologists in the United States. Fewer than a hundred of us specialize in prostate cancer. Defying all logic, medical oncologists are not trained in the treatment of early-stage prostate cancer to this day.

So how can a knowledgeable medical oncologist help a man with newly diagnosed prostate cancer? One of the biggest scientific breakthroughs has been the discovery that *we can make a clear distinction between the aggressive form of prostate cancer and the more common Low-Risk variety*. The latter form of the disease should probably not even be called cancer, but regarded instead as a *chronic condition*. This new awareness means that the surgical, one-size-fits-all way of thinking is both harmful and obsolete.

I have been treating men with prostate cancer for over fifteen years and my extensive experience is professional. I have never had an elevated PSA or undergone a prostate biopsy, nor have I experienced the hard choices that men with this disease must face. That is why this book would be incomplete without the testimony of a man who has personally lived through the ordeal of false cures, misinformation and risky invasive procedures. After twenty years of coexisting with the disease, his prostate still operational, my coauthor, Ralph Blum, is living proof that a diagnosis of prostate cancer is not automatically a death sentence. This book, then, is a collaboration between two experts, both with credentials, one on paper and one in the flesh.

The new information we have assembled in this book amounts to a road map to provide safe passage through a medical minefield. Research now shows that for most men surgery will not be beneficial, life is not prolonged and some degree of impotence or incontinence is almost guaranteed. What this book offers is the perspective of a cancer specialist intermixed in alternating chapters with a patient's firsthand experience navigating the treacherous medical terrain. Our aim is to present a better and more accurate way of thinking about prostate cancer that deals effectively with the disease and still preserves a man's quality of life.

1.

WELCOME TO PROSTATE COUNTRY

Just as there is an art to being a doctor, there is an art to being a patient.
You must choose wisely when to submit and when to assert yourself.

—ATUL GAWANDE, *Complications: Surgeon's Notes on an*
Imperfect Science

Prostate country is shadowy, misty territory, the Himalayas of masculine vulnerability. There are brigands lying in wait. And a shortage of reliable Sherpas. Although making the trek would not have been my personal choice, the experience has been profound, a midlife reeducation in taking responsibility (and at times *failing* to take responsibility) for decisions that affect your health, your well-being, your work in the world and, ultimately, your understanding of what it means to be a man.

The words "It's cancer," when spoken to you by a doctor, are among the most distressing in the language. To say that hearing them leaves you reeling would not be overstating it. And yet oddly, of all possible cancers, cancer of the prostate would be my cancer of choice. In fact, I am convinced that if the Lord of Hosts had appointed a committee of power hitters—the likes of Colin Powell, Michael Milken, General Schwarzkopf, Emperor Akihito and Arnold Palmer—to design a cancer especially for men, it would resemble the prostate cancer I have managed to coexist with for two decades.

The track I have followed has been scary at times, a cross between a high wire walk and a military exercise with live ammunition. When I was first diagnosed, the treatment options available today were still in the research stage. If they had been available back then, perhaps I might have made different choices. As it turned out, I became a contrarian, a renegade—someone who took up doctors' time asking questions and requiring explanations, and then refused to follow advice. What the Russians would call a "refusenik." Without realizing it, I suppose I turned into one of those feisty, difficult patients who, while irritating to doctors, often do well despite the odds. Or at least live quality lives for whatever time they have left.

THE EDUCATION OF A REFUSENIK

No one in my family or even among my close friends ever had cancer of the prostate, so it hadn't occurred to me that I might one day be diagnosed with the disease. In fact, I had never given any thought to that mysterious gland. However, once I joined the ranks of the newly diagnosed, I suddenly felt like I was standing in the middle of what Mark calls a medical minefield.

Here's how it usually goes: When your family doctor tells you that your PSA is above normal, or finds something "suspicious" while doing a DRE, he will refer you to a urologist who will—nineteen times out of twenty—perform a biopsy to determine whether the suspicious something is cancer. If cancer is confirmed, provided it is still contained within the prostate gland, and provided there is no medical reason surgery is counter-indicated, the urologist will almost certainly recommend it.

What the average guy—myself included—doesn't realize until that moment is that since the urologist is actually a surgeon, it's hardly surprising that his treatment of choice would be surgery. Aside from the fact that he genuinely believes surgery is your best option, there is the financial aspect. As one seasoned observer of the prostate cancer industry told me, "Your prostate is worth what Ted Turner would call 'serious cash money.'"

My own experience in the medical minefield began when Jeff Harris sent me to see Dr. Danforth. I knew next to nothing about the mechanics of a biopsy: how it works, how it could go wrong, what are the risks. It now appears that in my ignorance and my anxiety, I was less than fair to Dr. Danforth when I blamed him for blowing it. When I discussed that first biopsy with my old friend, Michael Klaper, MD, here's what he had to say:

No, he didn't "blow it." If the needle penetrates the tissue perpendicularly, and does not encounter anything but soft prostate tissue, the pathologist is given an intact core of tissue, relatively easy to read. But there may be a subtle curve to the surface that results in the needle penetrating slightly obliquely, which makes the forces upon the tissue going up the bore of the needle asymmetric, thus beginning to distort the shape of the core. If the needle then encounters a band of fibrous tissue, common enough in the prostate substance, a force will be exerted upon the core which further distorts it. Finally, if the already distorted core stubbornly refuses to come out of the needle, it must be extracted with an instrument, further changing the architecture — creating "crush artifact."

None of this is under the control of the urologist. Do this procedure on a thousand men, and it's a mathematical certainty that the process I have just described is going to happen to *someone*. In this case it was you. It's called being human.

Should I have been upset? Perhaps. In retrospect, I see that my overreaction was inappropriate and very risky. What if I'd had an aggressive form of prostate cancer? Waiting all those years before getting another biopsy might have been my death warrant.* Warning: I absolutely *do not* want to suggest that other men follow my potentially dangerous example. And yet, looking back, if it hadn't been for Dr. Danforth and crush artifact, my prostate cancer journey would probably have taken an entirely different course. What I first regarded as Dr. Danforth's botched biopsy actually bought me nine years of quality time during a period when "watchful waiting" (or the more military term "active surveillance") conflicted with the entire force and wisdom of the medical establishment.

INTRODUCING *HOMO UROLOGO*

If I was to avoid making a fool of myself again, I realized I needed a urologist I trusted as an advisor. I remembered my stepfather, Al Schwalberg, who had once been a federal agent, telling me years ago how, if a new cop in the New York Police Department wanted to get ahead, he needed a "rabbi," someone further up the ladder — almost certainly an Irishman — to mentor him and show him the ropes. What I needed was a prostate cancer rabbi. I found him in Larry Raithaus, MD, a urologist on the island of Kauai.

---

* Today there are less invasive ways to evaluate the aggressiveness of the cancer (see chapter 8), but at that time, biopsies were the only option.

I got to know Larry thanks to John Lilly, MD, the dolphin brain scientist, who rang me one day hoping that with my old LSD connections I might have access to a few cc's of ketamine, an animal tranquilizer used by some as a recreational drug, and, when injected intramuscularly, John's favorite "cocktail." I had no source for ketamine but I happened to have a painful kidney stone. So Lilly put me in touch with Raithaus, who hauled me over to St. Joseph's Hospital on Kauai for stone-blasting lithotripsy—and the beginning of a rewarding friendship.

After Michael Klaper had set me straight about the biopsy, I called Larry and asked him to brief me about the challenges a urologist faces.

"To begin with," Larry explained, "urologists are unique in that unlike all other surgeons, they also have a medical practice at least half of which involves dealing with problems like impotence, infections, incontinence and kidney stones. The average urologist has between twenty and thirty patients to see each day, in addition to operations to perform, reports to write, meetings to attend. He barely has time to keep up with what's new in his own field. And when your biopsy is positive, he has to make sure you understand all your treatment options, which usually calls for explaining, and then reexplaining. It takes a lot of time to educate a new patient. However, the average board-certified urologist knows that the law calls for 'informed consent.'"

"Meaning?"

"The law states that you have to present all viable treatment options. So I quote the stats on radiation, cryosurgery, and even explain about new treatments like proton beam therapy. I have my own list of experts in the field to whom I can refer patients for second and third opinions. I give them a lot of information and advice."

"Do they follow your advice?"

"That's the problem. Once they hear the word cancer, most of what I tell them after that won't even be absorbed. A lot of men will ask, 'What do *you* think, Doc? What would *you* do?' The average guy wants me to make the decision for him."

I told Larry that in my opinion there are two groups of men for whom surgery is unquestionably appropriate: first, those with an aggressive cancer that is still confined to the gland, and a second group—significantly larger—those men who, regardless of the nonthreatening character of their cancer, absolutely need to "just get it out!"

"That's fine, as long as the cancer complies with the surgeon's criteria for surgery," he said. "And believe me, even when it's Low-Risk disease, it's the rare man who's willing to wait, to just watch the cancer. Maybe one or two in a hundred will do what you're doing."

"One of the goals of the book Mark and I are writing," I told Larry, "is to encourage men with Low-Risk disease to think twice before rushing to make a radical treatment decision that is both unnecessary and likely to adversely affect the rest of their lives."

Larry said, "Fair enough. Those men can safely bide their time, provided they check their PSA and do follow-up ultrasounds. We watch for PSA doubling time. A PSA that doubles in less than three years is significant, and then a treatment decision has to be made sooner rather than later. In the end, it comes down to being an informed patient."

"How do you define an informed patient?"

He laughed, "Someone knowledgeable enough that he won't sue you."

My conversation with Larry left me feeling considerably more sympathetic about the challenges facing any urologist. He is the one, after all, who has to give you what is possibly the worst news of your life, educate you about the complexities of the disease and your treatment options, and help you manage the inevitable emotional trauma of the cancer diagnosis. In the end, I understood that it wasn't just the urologist who pushes for surgery. It was a combination of the urologist's preference for surgery and the "just get it out!" attitude of most men.

AND HERE'S YOUR OWN PERSONAL DEATH SENTENCE

Not all urologists are as diligent as Larry, or as compassionate.

After nine years, during which time my wife, Jeanne, and I explored a slew of complementary therapies and unorthodox treatment modalities, my PSA, which I had checked every three months, began creeping up. We were living on Maui when I finally submitted to a second biopsy with a urologist I'll call Dr. Garrison. It was less of an ordeal. It did, however, confirm cancer.

"Adenocarcinoma. Gleason score, 3 + 2," Dr. Garrison announced. He spoke in a flat voice, like he was reading a weather report. No preamble, no attempt to ease the blow. I sat there, silent, staring out the window at the tall palm trees swaying against the cloudless Maui sky, just trying to digest the fact that I did have cancer. Finally, he added, "You require surgery— now. You were very stupid to wait this long."*

Dr. Garrison was impatient and testy, the kind of doctor who wants nothing from a patient but compliance. He made no reference to other treatment options. When I told him I would think about his recommendation, he glared at me for a moment. Then he closed my file and growled, "Without surgery you'll be dead in two years."

I got up and left his office without saying a word.

For some time, I had suspected I had prostate cancer. Even with the uncertain diagnosis resulting from the crush artifact, the lump in my prostate was suspicious for cancer. But before hearing those grim words in Dr. Garrison's office, I had been feeling great and, strange to say, I hadn't been at all worried. I suppose my attitude was one of benign denial. The new biopsy results made the cancer real. But *dead in two years?* What I needed to know was how seriously to take Dr. Garrison's threat.

I was uncertain what to do next. Finally I decided to retrieve my slides from the pathologist on Maui and send them for a second opinion to Dr. David Bostwick, a respected pathologist who was at that time at the Mayo Clinic.

This, I now realize, was an important decision. Getting a second opinion on biopsy slides is always advisable, and virtually all insurance programs will cover the cost. The second opinion should preferably be given by a world-class reference center, such as Stanford, the Mayo Clinic or Johns Hopkins. Don't be afraid you will offend your doctor. Second opinion consultations are critical and they are standard procedure. If your doctor is offended, find another doctor.

FIRST DO NO HARM

When Dr. Garrison, in effect, sentenced me to death if I did not have surgery right away, he was violating the ancient medical precept incorporated

---

* The Gleason grading system assigns a grade to each of the two largest areas of cancer in the tissue samples from the biopsy. Grades range from 1 to 5, with 5 the most aggressive. The two grades are then added together to produce a Gleason Score. A Gleason Score of 2 to 10 is used to establish whether a prostate tumor is likely to be slow growing or aggressive: 2 to 6 is considered low grade; 7, intermediate grade; 8 to 10, high grade. So with a Gleason 3 + 2 my cancer was still in the low grade category, and Garrison's remark was uncalled for.

into the Hippocratic Oath taken by every doctor on graduating from medical school: *Primum non nocere.* "First do no harm."

A significant part of any doctor's job is to create a relationship with a patient based on trust, confidence and hope. Regardless of his knowledge or his experience, no physician can accurately predict how long a patient will live, nor does he have the right to do so. If you are advised by your doctor to "Go home and get your affairs in order," or told "There's nothing more I can do for you," and you are not a natural Refusenik, those words can do irreparable harm. At the very least, they amount to practicing prophecy without a license.

In his fine book, *Spontaneous Healing*, Andrew Weil, MD, called attention to "medical pessimism about the human potential for healing" and added, "At its most extreme, this attitude constitutes a kind of medical hexing that I find unconscionable . . . Although it is easy to identify this hexing phenomenon in exotic cultures, we rarely perceive that something very similar goes on every day in our own culture, in hospitals, clinics, and doctors' offices."

So what is the lesson here? Any time you are uncomfortable with your doctor, get a second opinion, and a third, and keep at it until you find someone you feel supports you in your healing process. Beware of the doctor who indulges in fear and hexing to influence your decisions. And if you ever do receive a "death threat," just remember: *That's his belief, not mine.* And head for the door.

THE PAVLOV EFFECT

The second opinion on the biopsy slides from Dr. Bostwick confirmed the diagnosis as "multiple foci of adenocarcinoma of the prostate," meaning there was cancer in a number of cores. Moreover, the Gleason score was raised to 3 + 3 = 6. Not what I wanted to hear. Yet I realize now that it was not such a big deal; a Gleason score of 6 is still in the *Low-Risk* category.

In spite of my unsettling experience with Dr. Garrison, I was still considering surgery. However, I was determined that if I was going to be cut open, I wanted it done at a major urban hospital and by a surgeon with whom I would feel totally secure. So I began scanning the field for surgeons with the best history of cure rates, like the pioneer of nerve sparing, Patrick Walsh at Johns Hopkins, Donald Skinner at USC, Peter Carroll at UCSF and Stuart Holden, Chief of Urology at Cedars Sinai in Los

Angeles. Obviously, the surgeon I was looking for was on the mainland. A month later, I flew to Los Angeles.

Shortly after my arrival in L.A., I had dinner with a friend, Jerry Moss, who offered to call Stuart Holden on my behalf. When I googled him, I found that Dr. Holden was also director of the Louis Warschaw Prostate Cancer Center and medical director of Michael Milken's Prostate Cancer Foundation (formerly Capcure), the largest private funder of prostate cancer research in the world. I gladly took Jerry up on his kind offer.

Dr. Holden made time to see me the next day. He was friendly and straightforward. The consult was brief. He looked at my history, asked me a few questions and then announced, "You're right for surgery. Talk to my secretary. There's room on my schedule next Thursday." And he was gone.

Enter the Refusenik. I never called his secretary. Nor did I even thank Dr. Holden for jumping me to the head of the line and offering me a place in his busy OR schedule. I was too embarrassed. I spent the next several days going over and over in my mind the reasons I was resisting surgery, despite the fact that having my prostate removed might give me my best shot at a cure. Finally, I called my cancer rabbi, Larry Raithaus, and told him what had happened. When Larry asked why I hadn't gone with Dr. Holden, I didn't know what to say. So I whined (this is so pathetic), "He didn't even do a *digital!*"

"Give me a break!" Larry said. "He had everything he needed to know in your records. Maybe if you'd *asked* him to do a DRE for *your* peace of mind, he would have. Listen, the guy is a black belt. He assumed, logically enough, that you had already decided on surgery when you came to see him. Why waste his time otherwise?

The question stayed with me: Why had I taken up Dr. Holden's time in the first place? I suppose, given my age, I was imprinted with the "surgery-is-the-gold-standard" propaganda of the prostate cancer culture that prevails to this day. I wasn't even considering other treatment options. Like one of Pavlov's dogs, I continued to salivate for a surgical solution. But after seeing Dr. Holden, and faced with the reality of surgery—actually being wheeled into the operating room *next Thursday!*—I freaked out. My mind was suddenly barraged by all the horror stories I'd heard about the collateral damage other guys had to live with after surgery.

What actually helped restore my perspective—or maybe it was my sanity—was remembering the opening of Vladimir Nabokov's novel, *Pnin*.

The author introduces his hero, Professor Timofei Pnin, who is riding comfortably through the countryside in a train compartment, and then goes on to describe him and his life in a full page of elaborate detail, right down to his socks which were "of scarlet wool with lilac lozenges." All of which, Nabokov finally admits, had nothing to do with the fact that Pnin was riding on the wrong train.

SAFE PASSAGE THROUGH THE MEDICAL MINEFIELD

Apart from my fear of the collateral damage from surgery, Jeanne and I were still hoping to have a baby. And if there's one thing that's certain it's no prostate, no baby. So for me, surgery was definitely "the wrong train."

Finding the courage to live with cancer is a no-holds-barred business, especially when it comes to knowing, as Atul Gawande aptly puts it, "when to submit and when to assert yourself," which is why I want to express my gratitude to those three very different urologists from whom I learned to give myself permission to be assertive.

From my experience with Dr. Danforth I learned that sometimes it's okay to make a decision based on instinct rather than reason. From Dr. Garrison I learned I was entitled to be angry at abusive authority. And from Dr. Holden I learned to give myself permission to say "No" when I felt that a procedure, even when performed by an expert, was not for me. Danforth-to-Garrison-to-Holden. *There's* a prostate cancer double play for you! My experience with each of the players contributed to my understanding that there is, indeed, an art to being a patient.

AND NOW MEET THE ENEMY

When you look at normal prostate tissue, you see how neat and well-formed the cells are, with a clear, sharply defined nucleus, healthy cytoplasm and cell membranes, all in an orderly arrangement and showing a healthy pink hue. As cancer advances from stage to stage, it starts to look less and less like its original cell type. The changes are the result of progression from a "well differentiated" cancer (less aggressive) to cells that are more aggressive or "poorly differentiated," which is to say they no longer resemble the parent cell line of normal prostate tissue cells. They have become darker, amorphous, with a shaggy outer membrane. Larry describes them as "evil bags of endlessly dividing protoplasm that will keep on dividing and dividing—deadly and immortal. Unless stopped."

RULE OF THUMB

If you have early stage prostate cancer—the indolent, Low-Risk kind that is about as threatening as mild chronic asthma—just be aware that mindless capitulation ("Whatever you say, Doc") can be dangerous. You have to make the big decisions for yourself. And bear in mind that the longer you can wait before you submit to *any* form of radical treatment, the better the odds that research in the field of prostate cancer will have advanced, and that treatment will have become more effective and less toxic.

Mark and I want to support you in finding your way safely through the medical minefield. What follows is a two-man show-and-tell, the result of an alliance between a prostate oncologist and his Refusenik patient. We will have accomplished what we set out to do if this book informs you, calms your fears, entertains you and leaves you with good reasons for hope.

THE DOCTOR'S VIEW

All patients seek caregivers who really care. How this obvious fact is lost on otherwise intelligent doctors constantly amazes me. Few things are more frightening than trusting your life to an impersonal and detached cancer specialist. The fact that Ralph has never been intimidated either by prostate cancer, or by doctors, has served him well through the years, allowing him to think clearly and form his own reasoned opinions. His decision to go slow, monitor the situation and take time to educate himself has given him many years of quality time with his wife that almost certainly would have been lost if he had committed to immediate surgery.

2.

ALL THE DECISION MAKERS ARE SURGEONS!

I believe that when the final chapter of this disease is written, it will
prove that never in the history of oncology will so many men have been
so over-treated for one disease.

—THOMAS STAMEY, MD,
Chief of Urology at Stanford University and developer of the PSA blood test

All doctors as healers, either consciously or subconsciously, develop a persona to create stability and inspire confidence. This is not all that different from an entertainer walking on stage who must catch and hold the audience's attention. Why? Because every patient has the option of gathering his belongings and moving on. A surgeon I know, Dr. Laura Cassidy, described it like this: "Every time you see a patient it has the intensity of a first date." If you're in private practice you want your clients to come back, so you treat them with the same care, energy and attention you would lavish on someone you're taking out for the first time.

You've heard of bedside manner? Well, let's dig below the surface and examine its origins and applications. A good bedside manner is not necessarily manipulative and self-serving; it can be helpful to the patient. A comforting demeanor is important for convincing patients to proceed with difficult or risky treatments when such treatments are truly required. A relationship between a doctor and a patient, a "therapeutic relationship," is based in one's faith and belief that the doctor can really help. In fact, in professional circles it is considered taboo to destroy a patient's trust in his doctor.

Ideally, men need to have some awareness of these realities *before* a doctor–patient relationship is established, that is to say, before a diagnosis of prostate cancer is made. Once you are diagnosed, it is entirely natural to look to your doctor to guide you through this alien and frightening terrain.

ONE EXAMPLE OF INAPPROPRIATE SURGERY

Let me illustrate how the magical attraction of "cutting it out" drives men toward ill-advised surgery even when they would be far better off selecting some other form of treatment. Not too long ago the vice president of a large firm consulted me for a second opinion about his recently diagnosed prostate cancer before proceeding with surgery. Steve is a tall, friendly sixty-seven-year-old man whom I had previously met a few times at church. Soon after he was diagnosed, he consulted with the chief of urology at the local university and scheduled an appointment for surgery. Steve's background in engineering led him to be particularly intrigued by theoretical advantages of the university's recently purchased da Vinci robot, a mechanical device that enables surgeons to operate through much smaller incisions than was previously possible.

After reviewing Steve's medical situation, I told him candidly that there were several other reasonable treatment alternatives and with all of them his survival would be at least as good as with surgery. In fact, in his case, long-term survival could be expected even if he underwent no immediate treatment at all. Then, as we delved further into his medical history, Steve mentioned a history of blood clots. "Yeah, when I was in my forties," he told me, "I almost died of a pulmonary embolism." Steve had been around doctors long enough to learn the technical term for a blood clot to the lung. Emboli can form in the legs or the large veins in the lower abdomen. When a clot breaks free and flows in the blood stream, it passes through the heart and lodges in the pulmonary artery, obstructing blood flow to the lungs. Blood can't get past the lungs to be oxygenated, so a large clot can result in asphyxiation. There were several other reasonable treatment options, so surgery for Steve was clearly contraindicated.

I bluntly shared my concerns with Steve. "Your history suggests a genetic predisposition to blood clots," I told him. "Prostate surgery would be particularly dangerous because the prostate is near the large veins of the pelvis where blood clots can form. If you have a congenital clotting problem, surgery will place you at high risk for another pulmonary embolism."

Much to my dismay, the surgeon and Steve went ahead with the scheduled operation anyway. Perhaps it was the temptation to use the new da Vinci robot. More likely it was the result of the urologist's deep conviction that surgery was in the patient's best interest.

I didn't hear about Steve's outcome until six weeks later when I was approached at church by his wife. "Mark, we feel so foolish," she confided in me. "Steve went ahead and had the operation and initially everything seemed to be going okay. But two weeks ago he suddenly started getting chest pains and became very short of breath. He was admitted to the hospital and put on blood thinners." She went on to tell me that there were some hairy moments where Steve's life hung in the balance but fortunately he survived the large clots to his lung. Later, after he went home from the hospital he consulted Donald Feinstein, MD, a hematologist at USC, who confirmed the diagnosis of a hereditary clotting abnormality and Steve was placed on long-term blood thinners.

Steve's case provides a disturbing example of the almost hypnotic sway that the quick fix of "cutting it out" holds over the minds of frightened men, even intelligent and accomplished men who have risen to the executive level in the business world.

INAPPROPRIATE SURGERY DOES NOT JUST "HAPPEN"

Before men decide on surgery, they go through a sequence of events starting with getting their PSA checked, and if it is elevated, seeing a urologist for a biopsy and, if the diagnosis is cancer, undergoing treatment. During this sequence, a critically important moment of decision usually passes without adequate consideration. A decision to do surgery is often made without the patient realizing how biased his surgeon-advisor is in favor of operating. Men don't realize that through experience and practice, doctors develop a persuasive, soft-sell approach; everything about their demeanor and body language conveys the message that surgery is the best treatment. Most men never understand these dynamics until it's too late. This entire process begins to unfold when you hear your family doctor say, "Your PSA is elevated and I am referring you to a urologist. He may want to do a biopsy."

This is the moment when you need to take a breath and say you'd like to do some research before taking the next step rather than rushing forward. In the course of this book we will consider what that next step should be.

The implications of starting your potential cancer journey with a surgeon at the helm should at least give you pause. Most men are unaware of the chain of events that will follow if a biopsy reveals the presence of cancer. And yet studies show that microscopic amounts of low-grade prostate cancer are so common *that even when the PSA is totally normal, one-fourth of men will have a positive biopsy!*[1] So if the biopsy *is* positive, it is assumed that the urologist will take over your prostate cancer care. When does the patient discover this? *After the biopsy* when the urologist calls and says, "It's cancer" and recommends that a time be booked for surgery.

Assume you've just learned that you have prostate cancer. As an uninformed lay person, you reckon your demise is imminent. All of a sudden you're on death row. Your wife and children will agonize about losing the most important man in their lives. Your friends will look at you differently. So will your insurance company.

Now factor in your own shock and horror, the unbalancing and disorienting realization that you have cancer. You have just received what is possibly the worst news of your life. The psychological impact of a cancer diagnosis is overwhelming. Only moments before you were a normal healthy person. Suddenly, you are flooded with feelings of grief and terror. Rational thought is gone; emotion takes over. A newly diagnosed cancer patient is like a newborn duckling yet to be imprinted on its mother. After diagnosis, you are born into a new and uncertain world. And there is no way to go back.

Under these pressured circumstances the urologist smoothly assumes leadership. He seizes the wheel and you become the passenger. Disoriented, you have no idea, no idea at all, of what you have just done. You have become one more dutiful lamb being herded into the pen. You've already had one intimate experience with this stranger. You have already trusted him by allowing him to poke needles into what one woman called "the true heart of the male." Why wouldn't you trust him now to prescribe his treatment of choice? It simply doesn't occur to you to think otherwise. The hook has been set. What usually happens is that you will uncritically proceed to make an appointment for surgery.

Before you consult a urologist to have a biopsy performed you should consider the following question, "Do you really want a surgeon to advise you on whether or not surgery is indicated?" Don't we already know what treatment the urologist is going to prescribe? Biopsy itself is not particularly dangerous but the psychological impact of a cancer diagnosis is monumental.

Consider a parallel situation that many of us are familiar with: going into a car dealership to buy a car. Most of us know that a car salesman is skilled at what he does, that he will try to portray himself as a trustworthy friend. Ignorant people who accept this "friendship" at face value suffer severely in the wallet. Even when we know what to expect, the car salesman still has a huge advantage. After all, he has what you want. In a sense the urologist is in the exact same position because you are definitely in the market for a cure.

When your PSA is elevated, or your DRE is suspicious, your family doctor will refer you to a urologist to have a biopsy performed. However, I suggest that before you take that first step, it's important to take the time to do some research. An immediate biopsy may not be in your best interest. (The question of how to determine if a biopsy is necessary is addressed in more detail in chapter 8.) Although I am absolutely in favor of doing a biopsy when it is appropriate, one of the reasons I agreed to write this book with Ralph was my concern over the number of unnecessary biopsies performed—not to mention the number of unnecessary surgeries that follow.

THE "JUST CUT IT OUT" SCHOOL OF PROSTATE CANCER

The emotional appeal of "cutting it out" can even sway medical professionals who should know better. George Rinaldi, age seventy-five, was himself a retired general surgeon. Like Steve, he was already sold on the idea of surgery with the da Vinci robot when he came to me for a second opinion on his early-stage cancer. He was intrigued by the thought that the operation would be less risky because the skin incisions are substantially smaller.

"Dr. Rinaldi," I told him, "I know with your training and background, surgery looks like an attractive option. But given your age you should consider another alternative such as radiation, cryotherapy or testosterone deprivation."

I explained that even the urology textbooks cite the risks of surgery in the elderly. Patrick Walsh, inventor of nerve-sparing prostate surgery and one of the world's most eminent urologists, is adamant about not operating on any man over a certain age. His standard joke is that he will not do surgery on someone over seventy unless both parents accompany him to the consultation, the point being that early-stage prostate cancer grows too slowly to cause mortality within ten years.[2] If this is your situation, then why endure the risks and side effects of a major surgical procedure?

Five months after my initial consultation with Dr. Rinaldi my secretary informed me that I had a phone call.

"Mark, this is George Rinaldi."

"Hi, how are you doing? What treatment did you finally select?"

"That's why I'm calling you," he said hesitantly. "I went ahead with the surgery."

"How did it go?"

"Not well. It was complicated by massive blood loss. During the operation I was transfused with fifteen units of blood. After the surgery the wound became infected so they started me on antibiotics. The antibiotics caused a severe diarrhea that has taken months to recover from. But that's not the worst of it. I had a colostomy."

"A colostomy! How did that happen?"

"The surgery caused a vesiculorectal fistula." (A vesiculorectal fistula is an abnormal passageway between the rectum and the bladder.) "I made the diagnosis on myself on the third day after surgery . . ."

Dr. Rinaldi seemed to hesitate. So I said, "What prompted your diagnosis?"

"I farted through my penis."

"You *what!*"

"Yeah, well, it may sound like a joke, but it sure wasn't funny. It was really painful. They tried to close the opening with another operation. When that failed they had to do the colostomy. But that's not the reason I'm calling. They want to do another surgery to reverse the colostomy but I thought I'd better consult you first."

I told him to make an appointment to see me. What worried me was that if he underwent another surgery, the doctors would need to restart antibiotics. After a case of severe antibiotic diarrhea, retreatment is almost certain to reactivate the diarrhea.

Dr. Rinaldi came into the office the following week. Considering what he had been through he looked good. When I complimented him, he said, "Since the diarrhea stopped last month I've been able to regain some of the weight I lost."

After reviewing his case I offered my advice.

"The risk I see with another operation is that more antibiotics will be needed. Please don't proceed without consulting an infectious disease specialist. Even a small exposure to antibiotics would almost certainly reactivate the diarrhea."

I sent a copy of my consultation to his surgeon, expressing my concerns in no uncertain terms.

By now you can probably guess where this story is going. The surgeon could not be derailed from doing another operation. No infectious disease doctor was consulted. Dr. Rinaldi underwent another operation. The diarrhea came back and again took several months to resolve.

Men under the gun of a cancer diagnosis are emotionally vulnerable. Superior intelligence, even medical training, is not enough to counter the disorienting effect of being dumped into the emotional vortex of a new prostate cancer diagnosis. Both Steve and Dr. Rinaldi had gone the extra mile by consulting an outside expert (me) regarding the advisability of doing surgery. They had wisely selected a large referral center rather than having surgery with a community urologist.* Despite this, both Steve and Dr. Rinaldi were poor candidates for surgery and both nearly paid with their lives.

SO WHAT'S AT STAKE HERE?

Surgeons are members of a very select fraternity. They have made a huge personal investment in learning how to perform the complex surgical procedure known as the radical prostatectomy. Their genuine belief that surgery provides the best chance for cure makes their arguments extremely compelling. However, an operation needs a willing partner. In shock, the newly diagnosed man fails to consider the impact of losing potency and normal urinary function in the rush to do surgery. It is only after the surgery that the reality of sexual incapacity sets in.

Studies show that impotence totally redefines a man's self-esteem, his self-confidence and relational satisfaction.[3] And contrary to popular belief, Viagra does not correct surgically induced impotence. Penis vacuum devices, penis tourniquets, penis injections (yes with needles) or the surgical implantation of a plastic rod into the penis itself is often required to restore function. These devastating realities are often glossed over by the surgeon.

---

* Peter Bach, MD, in the *Wall Street Journal*, October 27, 2007, page A9, reports: "In New York State in 2002, the average prostate surgeon performed fewer than four operations, and there were 114 surgeons who did only one prostate operation." In the U.S. there are somewhere around 50,000 radical prostatectomies done annually, and there are 10,000 urologists. If you do the math it's clear that the average community urologist can't be doing enough prostate surgery to stay proficient.

In the 1990s, the only alternatives to surgery were castration or unfocused toxic radiation. But with the advent of new drugs, testosterone blocking can be reversible (chapter 10). Modern radiation is both less toxic and more effective than surgery (chapter 12). Yet many radiation therapists hesitate to tell this to their patients for fear such comments will get back to the referring urologist. Far too often I see radiation therapists recommending surgery even though they know that a well-performed radioactive seed implant has comparable if not superior cure rates.[4,5,6] This happens because the radiation therapists want to keep their referral pipeline from the urologists open. After all, they know there will be future referrals they can treat—such as older men who are poor surgical candidates—as long as they keep in the good graces of the urologists. The unspoken tenet is: "Radiation for the elderly and surgery for the rest."

I don't believe that mere business concerns fuel urologists' propensity for surgery. Rather it is the huge personal investment they make in learning how to perform this complex operation. They work hard to get to medical school and generally they rise to the top of their classes. Surgical training requires long hours and sleepless nights with incessant pressure and competition. However, because of all this, they often lack objectivity when giving advice about the need for surgery.

To sum up: When a family doctor refers you to a urologist, your first line of defense is to be aware of the awesome implications of rushing into a prostate biopsy. The second line of defense, if a biopsy has already been performed, is to refrain from undergoing an irreversible treatment until the emotion of the situation wears off and you have had time to carefully analyze all the circumstances. As you will see, Ralph's experiences throughout the book exemplify an attitude of caution and patience, an attitude that has led to good decision making. Thankfully, as will be clearly seen in my next chapter, prostate cancer is slow growing—there is no reason to rush. Rushing leads to bad decisions.

THE PATIENT'S VIEW

Mark's reference to "imprinting" is very astute, evoking for me the picture of Konrad Lorenz followed by a train of newly hatched graylag goslings. The physician becomes our "parent" in matters of trust.

We really don't need or want to have to think about every piece of advice or decision. *Can I trust this guy?* must not be among the questions that trouble our newly diagnosed selves. When I heard from one urologist that he is comfortable doing *ninety-six unnecessary surgeries* in order to save two lives, I began having "what is wrong with this picture?" thoughts. And then I learned that for a surgeon to be up to speed with the new robotic technologies, it takes 250 practice attempts. I can just hear myself, as I am going under the anesthetic, remembering to ask, "By the way, Doc, where am I in your learning curve?"

3.

THE QUEST FOR AN ENCHANTED SHOTGUN

Remember to check the unusual stuff that's out there. Some of it
has real merit. And don't forget that enjoyment of life is part of the
treatment. Have some good times. Guys who go to Florida and Arizona
do better. There's a lot more to this disease than meets the eye.

—BILL BLAIR

The nine years bracketed by my first two biopsies were spent in "Paradise." Shortly after my run-in with Dr. Danforth, Jeanne and I moved from Malibu to Maui. We bought a lovely old plantation house in the village of Haiku and ran it as a bed and breakfast. Life in upcountry Maui has got to be good for whatever ails you. We grew our own vegetables, swam with giant turtles and dolphins, took long walks on sandy beaches and quiet country roads where the only illumination at night came from the moon and the stars. The pace was leisurely, life was sweet and somehow I didn't worry much about prostate cancer. Still, I got regular checkups and tracked my PSA, which didn't seem to be going anywhere.

TRADITIONAL ORIENTAL MEDICINE

However, I did not go untreated. Through all those years, I had the good fortune to be living with my therapist wife, Jeanne, herself a cancer survivor and a skilled practitioner of Traditional Oriental Medicine (TOM). Soon after the "crush artifact" biopsy, she began giving me weekly acupressure treatments in her specialty, auricular therapy (from the Latin, *auricula*, the ear), one of the oldest branches of Chinese medicine.

Because all the body's energy flows (meridians) meet in the ear, Jeanne treats the entire body through 365 tiny points along the surface of each ear. She does not needle or pierce the skin. She uses a small hand-held tool made of bone and tipped with gold on one end to stimulate a point, and with silver on the other end to sedate or tone the energy down. In the case of my prostate point, it was always the gold tip, so that the prostate was stimulated to release its unhealthy energy.

When Jeanne was giving me an ear treatment, she would work any point that needed balancing (liver, spleen, kidneys), always ending with the prostate. When she began to work the prostate point, I would experience considerable tenderness and pain in that spot on my ear, but that would gradually diminish as the negative energy was released. For most auricular therapists, the release occurs independent of the practitioner. In Jeanne's case, the toxic energy exits through *her* body. Quite often, while working my prostate point, she would look pale and feel nauseated. On several occasions she almost vomited. These sessions would last up to two hours and required a very steady hand to hold the tiny tool accurately on the point until the release was completed.

I am making no recommendations with respect to auricular therapy as a treatment option for cancer. I am simply reporting my experience. Yet I am convinced that Jeanne's regular ear treatments contributed substantially to our successful two decades of prostate cancer management.

WHAT'S IN A NAME? "ALTERNATIVE" VERSUS "COMPLEMENTARY"

Energy work is just one of many healing modalities that are found under the umbrella of "alternative" medicine. Whereas conventional medicine relies primarily on surgery, radiation and drugs to treat disease, alternative medicine calls on the body's own healing powers to manage illness. However, the term "alternative" seems to imply an either/or approach to treatment choices. "Complementary" medicine, on the other hand, describes an approach that, rather than attempting to replace mainstream medical treatments, seeks to take advantage of any technique that contributes to and supports a patient's overall healing protocols and wellness.

The field of alternative medicine is vast, and includes a wide range of therapies. At one end of the spectrum you will find therapies that complement conventional treatment. These would include herbs, botanicals, nutritional supplements, acupuncture and acupressure, aromatherapy and various forms of massage including although not limited to reflexology, shiatsu and Reiki, as well as visualization, guided imagery, affirmations, meditation and relaxation techniques. At the more extreme end of the spectrum, you will find the mysterious Rife machine, Brazilian psychic surgeons and various other intriguing but questionable methods of healing.

Maui proved to be a veritable Shangri-La for unconventional treatment modalities, a caravan stop for healers from all over the world. Finding myself in a no-man's-land of diagnostic uncertainty, I was curious to know what options were out there. So during the nine years Jeanne and I lived on Maui, I subjected myself to a number of unorthodox treatments, almost all of which operate beneath the FDA radar.

A lot of people are looking for a single magic bullet. I decided I'd settle for an enchanted shotgun. What follow are some of the farther-out areas I explored.

CESIUM CHLORIDE

If you consult "Dr. Google" about cesium chloride as a cancer treatment, you will come up with more than 20,000 results. However, while there are some interesting case studies, the documented evidence is murky. And while the American Cancer Society recognizes the use of cesium-137 in certain types of radiation therapy, it is no fan of cesium chloride as a "High pH Cancer Therapy."

The therapeutic use of cesium chloride (CsCl), a salt form of cesium-137, is mainly the result of research by Aubrey Brewer, PhD (1893–1986), and is based on the theory that cancer cells thrive in an acidic environment but perish in an alkaline, high pH environment. Cesium chloride supposedly works by raising the cancer cell's pH to a highly alkaline, and therefore deadly, state.

Despite the American Cancer Society's position that "available scientific evidence does not support this theory," there is a considerable market for cesium chloride in the Enchanted Shotgun Derby, and there is plenty of product available. When I began my research, it was being administered intravenously, nasogastrically and orally. I decided to take cesium chloride orally for six weeks as a cleanse.

I can't judge whether in my case the cesium chloride had any cancer-retarding effects. I can say, however, that the stuff was quite disgusting and made me feel sick. So I stopped taking it after two weeks. Maybe I was just chicken. But I was still learning, as they say, to listen to my body, and like the American Cancer Society—and my writing partner— my body was no fan of cesium chloride.

OZONE THERAPY: THE COMMON MAN'S HYPERBARIC CHAMBER

According to Dr. Otto Warburg, who won the Nobel prize for his research into cellular respiration and cancer, cancer cells can readily form and thrive in a low or depleted oxygen environment. The theory behind ozone therapy is that while healthy cells are aerobic and need oxygen to survive, unhealthy cells, bacteria and viruses are anaerobic and can only survive in the absence of oxygen. In other words, as the theory goes, cancer cells cannot exist in a high oxygen environment. However, apparently ozone "peroxydizes" lung tissue, meaning that it is toxic enough to destroy sensitive tissue. So don't breathe it, right? Still, the idea that a technique for cleansing your blood can prove fatal is, to say the least, somewhat daunting.

Several upcountry Maui therapists were administering IV infusions of ozone (O_3). The procedure involved removing a small quantity of blood from the body, placing it in an infusion bottle, saturating it with oxygen and then returning the oxygen-rich blood back into the body. However, my friend, Billy Driver, a biochemist and himself a prostate cancer survivor, warned me: "Ozone is like a razor blade: you can shave with it, and you can use it to cut your throat."

Although proponents claim that ozone therapy is safe and nontoxic as long as it's administered responsibly, I decided I didn't want anyone messing with my blood. So when I learned that I could receive the ozone transdermally (through the skin's surface), I allowed myself to be zipped into a body bag—a black plastic affair known locally as an "ozone sauna suit" that was connected by a hose to an ozone tank. The treatments were scheduled weekly, lasted about half an hour and seem to have had no adverse side effects.

Ozone therapy, although popular in Europe for many years, is still considered an untrustworthy treatment by the American Cancer Society. To this day, I still have no idea whether the few treatments I had did me any good. Still, as I lay there listening to the sibilant hiss of the ozone surrounding my

body and passing through my skin, I made an effort to visualize all the itin-
erant pathogens and damaged or infected cells snorting the gas and going
belly up, which, in turn, encouraged me to believe that the ozone treatment
I was getting was indeed protecting my body from harm.

PC-SPES: CUTTING CORNERS IN THE NAME OF "HOPE"

I liked the cool acronym, which stands for "Prostate Cancer—Hope," (*spes*
being Latin for "hope") because hope is what the herbal compound gave
thousands of men with advanced prostate cancer. Based on a Chinese
herbal formula, PC-SPES drove down elevated PSAs, decreased testosterone levels, lowered blood pressure and attacked prostate cancer cells. Published studies documented the product's effectiveness, and clinical trials,
begun in the 1990s, reported that it slowed the growth of prostate cancer.
In fact PC-SPES looked like a viable, reasonably priced, readily available
herbal form of hormone blockade with side effects like breast enlargement
and decreased libido to prove it.

Then the problems began.

It turned out that along with the eight listed Chinese herbs, PC-
SPES was found to contain a variety of undeclared prescription drug
ingredients—estrogen, warfarin (a blood thinner), and alprazolam, also
known as Xanax—which, if present in sufficient quantities and not taken
under medical supervision, *might* cause health problems. However, the
amounts were deemed by some to be too small to be consequential, and
it was never determined whether their inclusion was by the manufacturer or one of the suppliers.

After I took PC-SPES for a short time, my PSA started to drop. I believed I had found a winner and I stocked up with a good supply. So it
came as a shock when the news of possible adulteration broke and the
manufacturer, Botanic Lab, voluntarily recalled the product. Since then,
I have talked to men who still swear by PC-SPES, are convinced they
benefited mightily from taking it, even owe their lives to it and were extremely upset by the recall. Once PC-SPES was no longer commercially
available, a black market for the drug sprang up complete with vendors
who operated like scalpers selling tickets to Broadway shows. I was offered
up to $200 for a month's supply, for which I had paid only $50. Speculate
in PC-SPES futures? Bad idea.

Then an interesting thing happened. Although PC-SPES is no longer legal in the U.S., there is a thriving business that sprang up in Hong Kong and produced a similar product. While working on this chapter, I received an unsolicited call from the proprietor, Larry Pope, doing a hard sell, grabbing my attention with, "In three months you're gonna be dead if you don't order this product!" Seems he was talking about a version of PC-SPES, renamed CancerSpes in its new incarnation. Mr. Pope proceeded to tell me he had saved the lives of 36,000 men, and ordered me to call a certain Doc Lane. "He'll set you straight," he assured me.

Dead in three months . . . Now there's a promotional message for you! If he was right, I'd be toast long before this book was published. I marked the date on my calendar.

Out of curiosity, I rang Doc Lane, whose first question to me was, "Are you a man of faith?" And when I answered in the affirmative, he said, "Larry has saved me three times. Order the product, do what he tells you to do and move forward. He doesn't sell to anyone he cannot help. I speak as a man of God. I gotta run." And Doc Lane took another call.

Mr. Pope had moved his operation from Alabama to Hong Kong. When I checked, I found him on Dr. Google where he listed his new company as LarryCancerSpes. From Hong Kong, the product was shipped to L.A., then trucked to Alabama and from there distributed to buyers. A month's supply (with shipping) cost $450, or about the price of a week's holiday in Cancun.

In our last conversation, Mr. Pope claimed that "a month will usually take care of any cancer." So do the math. Even if his 36,000 customers only went for a single month's supply, that's a gross of over sixteen million dollars. Add Brother Pope to the roster of men who have "benefited mightily" from PC-SPES.

PROMISING BUT NOT YET MAINSTREAM:
LIGHT THERAPY AND HYPERTHERMIA

A friend invited me to attend an evening lecture on light therapy. The speaker, a PhD from Germany, explained that light therapy was first practiced in the ancient Greek city of Heliopolis, the city of the sun, famous for its healing temples. Today, light therapy, aka photodynamic therapy (PDT), works by employing a photosensitizing agent that is injected into the bloodstream. The agent is absorbed by all the cells but remains longer in cancer cells. Approximately twenty-four to seventy-two hours after the injection, when most of the agent has left the normal cells, light is directed into the body through fiber optic cables to the area of the tumor. The photosensitizing agent in the tumor absorbs the light and produces oxygen that destroys nearby cancer cells. In 2009 seven hospitals in the U.K. were offering the treatment, and TV personality Sir David Frost was so impressed by the experience of a friend treated with photodynamic therapy for the return of a mouth tumor that he agreed to help raise £50 million to fund research.

Up to now, PDT has been used primarily to treat head and neck cancers, but clinical trials are currently under way in the U.S. to evaluate its use with other cancers, including prostate cancer. In addition to killing cancer cells, PDT is said to destroy the blood vessels that feed cancer cells in the tumor. Proponents claim that this treatment can also activate the immune system to attack tumor cells.

Hyperthermia (doc-speak for high temperature) has been used to treat cancer since the early 1970s, based on the premise that cancer cells are more susceptible to extreme heat than normal healthy cells. Research has shown that super-high temperatures (up to 113° Fahrenheit) increase the flow in the lymphatic system by eighteen times, which may help to explain the role of hyperthermia, or "artificial fever," in cancer therapy. To ensure that the desired temperature is reached but not exceeded, the temperature of the tumor and surrounding tissue is carefully monitored during treatment.

Several methods of hyperthermia are currently under study including local, regional and whole-body (for metastatic cancer). In local hyperthermia, heat can be applied by microwave, radiofrequency and ultrasound. In regional perfusion, some of the patient's blood is removed, heated and then pumped (perfused) back into the limb or organ. Whole-body hyperthermia can include the use of hot water blankets or thermal chambers similar to large incubators.

This treatment has been used in Germany for years. Here in the U.S., a number of clinical trials have shown mixed results. The procedure is mostly used in combination with conventional cancer treatments, such as radiation therapy.

Parmenides, a Greek physician (540–480 B.C.) allegedly said, "Give me the power to produce fever and I can heal every illness." It occurred to me that if you want to live dangerously, you can obtain similar results by giving the patient malaria and then curing it. Could you, I wondered, cleanse cancer cells from the blood by sending the temperature soaring? Perhaps if I had advanced prostate cancer, I'd be a willing volunteer. As things stood, I'd have to say, "Hold the hyperthermia!"

THE MYSTERIOUS RIFE MACHINE

Invented in the 1930s by Dr. Royal Raymond Rife, the Beam Ray Machine, aka the Rife Machine, is considered by some a giant in the annals of medical quackery or, at best, a Walter Mitty experience. Rife himself was accused by the American Medical Association of fraudulent medical practices. However, there are those who believe he was a genius, and claim that his device helps people with a wide range of conditions from yeast infections and arthritis to Parkinson's and cancer.

Rife discovered he could use specific electromagnetic frequencies to kill bacteria and viruses without damaging healthy cells or surrounding tissue. His machine relies on what he called "sympathetic resonance" to physically vibrate the cells of a parasite until the vibration is intense enough to destroy the targeted cells, perhaps in much the same way as a high musical note can shatter a wine glass, or ultrasound can be used to destroy gallstones.

I spent many sun-drenched afternoons on Maui hooked up to a new version of the Rife Machine at the house of Spencer Feldman, a technical wizard and alternative treatment maven. I would sit in a comfortable chair wrapped in a loose garb of wire coils—a cross between a Buck Rogers bassinet and a stripped-down Faraday cage—listening to humming noises and watching pulsing lights as the machine did its thing. Spencer told me there had been good results reported with colon, skin and lung cancers.

"The machine goes after a virus that may or may not be causing a cancer," he explained. "If you don't have that virus, it's not going to do anything."

"That sounds pretty indefinite," I said.

"You want definite?" said Spencer. "Even if it doesn't cure you, it's definitely not going to do you any harm."

There is considerable doubt about the efficacy of the Beam Ray Machine, but there is no doubt that Royal Rife experienced hard times in the Land of Opportunity. During the latter part of his life, he was apparently subjected to all kinds of harassment by both the U.S. government and witch hunt–prone citizens. And yet his machine soldiers on. New incarnations of the Rife Machine can be purchased on the Internet. One ergonomically up-market version is currently available at a discount price of $1,795. You pay the shipping.

"DR. FRITZ IS COMING TO TOWN"

My friend Billy Driver always knew what was happening allopathically and alternatively on the island. One December morning, I got a dawn call from him, waking me up with, "Rise and shine, Blum! Dr. Fritz, the new boss psychic surgeon is coming to town! The line is already forming."

The so-called psychic surgeons of Brazil and the Philippines first came to my attention when an old friend, Andrija Puharich, MD, went to Brazil to study José Arigo, best known as "the surgeon with a rusty knife." Arigo performed unusual feats of surgery without sterilized instruments or anesthesia, and claimed he served as a conduit for the spirit of a dead German surgeon, Dr. Adolfo Fritz. Puharich spent months with Arigo during which time he witnessed and filmed hundreds of operations, including the removal of a benign tumor from his own arm using an unsterilized penknife. According to Puharich, the procedure lasted barely fifteen seconds and there was no anesthetic, no pain, almost no bleeding, no wound that required stitches and no post-op infection.

In the rarefied world of psychic surgery, the Brazilian, Joao Teixeira de Faria, aka "John of God," is a very big deal indeed. You can check him out on YouTube and the Discovery Channel. ABC's *Primetime* produced an hour-long show about him that aired February 12, 2005. Thanks to John of God, an entire industry has sprung up, attracting droves of people to Casa de Dom Ignacio, John of God's "energetic hospital" in the tiny village of Abadiania in central Brazil. Not including airfare, one typical guided tour costs about $1,500 and promises "twelve sessions with the entity." At one time, Dr. Fritz was John of God's "main healing spirit." Then business exploded, and today John of God claims that he channels more than thirty "doctor entities" who are all, one might say, "board certified" in the spirit surgery world.

That morning, Billy told me that Rubens Faria, a Brazilian computer engineer who also "channeled" Dr. Fritz, would be on Maui for a week.

I decided to get in line and see for myself what this bizarre phenomenon was all about.

It was a cloudy Saturday morning just before Christmas. My appointment with Rubens was for 9:00 AM up in Olinda at the house where Billy was living. There were two or three people ahead of me, so I sat outside on the porch until it was my turn. Mourning doves were pecking in the scrub grass and a small boy was swinging in a tire suspended from a branch of a banyan tree, the rubbing rope making a creaking sound. Although I believe that miracle cures can occur, as I sat there I wondered: *How do you tell the real thing from the false?*

"Ralph, come in."

Rubens Faria stood holding the screen door open and smiling. A slender man somewhere in his forties, wearing a short-sleeved white shirt and white duck trousers, he didn't offer to shake hands. He gestured for me to sit on a massage table covered with an orange and green cloth, and asked, "How can I help?"

I was skeptical and reluctant to even mention my prostate. Instead, I pointed to a lipoma I'd had for years, a small squidgy lump on the brow ridge just above my left eyebrow and said, "This is something I have no use for."

Rubens probed the lipoma gently with two fingers and said in German, "*Warum nicht?*" Why not?

I was somewhat reassured by the shirt he was wearing—nothing up his sleeves! Still, I kept my eyes open, watching, I admit, for any tricks. Rubens (or was it now Dr. Fritz?) placed one hand supportively behind my head; the other hand was lightly touching the flesh over my left eye. All I felt was a slight pinching sensation. Then he said, "*Gut gemacht!*" which I took to mean, "Well done."

After only a few seconds he released my head. Then he was dabbing at my forehead with a blue bandanna. He showed me, in his open palm, what appeared to be a small blob of fat surrounded by the remains of what might have been membrane. I wish now that I had asked for the blob as a souvenir—and to show to a pathologist. But I was probably in an altered state of my own by then. So I just thanked Rubens, and placed a donation in a bowl on a stand by the door.

As I was leaving, I turned and said, "I do have one question. Do you feel what you're doing is, well, the future of medicine?"

The only sound was the creaking of the rope made by the child swinging in the tire. Rubens smiled. "The medicine of the future," he said quietly, "will be the medicine of love."

A few weeks later, when I reported my experience with Rubens to my cancer rabbi, Larry snorted and said, "I don't believe it for a minute."

"There's a concave spot where the lipoma used to be," I said defensively.

"You can crush a fatty tumor with your fingers."

"But I didn't feel any pressure. And besides," I added, playing my trump card, "there's even a scar."

"A small scar is easy. It doesn't go deeper than the epidermis."

Obviously Larry and Rubens came from different medical traditions. I am reminded of something St. Ignatius Loyola once said: "For those who believe, proof is unnecessary. For those who do not believe, no proof is possible." Then again, if I remember correctly, Loyola was talking about salvation.

In my files, I have a photograph of "Dr. Fritz," aka Rubens, treating a patient in London. Along Rubens' right side you can see a shadow-image extending from his scalp down to his fingers. The woman who sent me the picture appended this note: "Obviously a double exposure, or an artifact from the development process. Still, the 'true believers' insist that the shadow is evidence of an appearance by the elusive Dr. Fritz."

By now, over 800,000 people have sought help from Rubens Faria at his clinic in a suburb of Rio de Janeiro. I can't help wondering: Is it possible to deceive that many people? Perhaps I should have let Dr. Fritz have a go at my prostate.

JUST ANOTHER BOTTLE LABELED "DRINK ME!"

Once you start on this quest, it's hard to quit. I've kept at it throughout my years of living with prostate cancer. Before I leave this chapter, I want to tell you about the most recent source of ammunition for the Enchanted Shotgun, something called "the APeX Solution," a treatment regarded by most of my friends as about as sensible as placing a bet on a three-legged horse.

In May of 2008 I started taking a teaspoon of the Solution twice a day in eight ounces of water. Colorless, odorless, tasteless, it caused me no discomfort, unless I count a mild sense of guilt because I was self-medicating again with an unproved substance, and doing so without conferring with my oncologist/coauthor.

According to the manufacturer, the APeX Research Institute, I was drinking a "silver and oxygen solution" described somewhat obliquely on the bottle as "silver atoms permanently bonded to multiple oxygen atoms in atomic chain units at a subnanological unit size of 0.33 nanometers in purified water." Dumb that down and it translates roughly as silver particles small enough to be transported across cell walls. So who takes this concoction? Mostly people with advanced cancer and AIDS, people who have given up hope. Providing you join an ICAM (Integrative Complementary & Alternative Medicine) study, the APeX Research Institute will, as of this writing, provide you with a regular supply of the Solution *free of charge*. That alone makes it stand out in the field of money-driven medicine.

Nota bene: APeX has not yet been submitted for FDA approval. No phase I, II and III tests have been run. There's no guarantee of the Solution's effectiveness or of its down-range safety. (Ten years from now my nose may fall off!) So I want to be clear that I'm making no claim of scientific value for what I'm reporting here. Nor is my experience meant to encourage anyone to follow my track.

Since antiquity, however, silver has been used to fight disease and promote healing. Contemporary studies have shown that silver is a potent enough antibacterial agent to be used extensively in burn units, operating rooms, and even to have served in a water purification system on the NASA space shuttle. As someone said, "Silver is worth its weight in gold."

In late February 2008, before embarking on my own phase I test of the APeX Solution—with myself as the sole study subject—I went to Duke Bahn for a color Doppler ultrasound in order to establish a baseline. Five months later I went back to Ventura for a repeat ultrasound. Interpreting the test results, and without any prompting from me, the Duke remarked that there was one unexpected change in my status: there was no new blood flow to my tumor. "No appreciable neovascularity" was the phrase he entered in his report.

During this period the only medication I was taking was Avodart (see Appendix). But I had already been taking Avodart daily for over a year, with no reduction of blood flow. In my latest ultrasound in November of 2009, there was still no new blood flow to the tumor.

When I finally showed the APeX material to Mark, who has been reasonably tolerant of my continuing quest for the Enchanted Shotgun, he shrugged and said, "Well, you're the guy who's willing to pan for gold in the 1% mine." He then reminded me of a point he makes in chapter 20: that in our modern information age, *truly effective remedies* never remain obscure for very long. "When they work," he said, "they jump right to the top of the charts."

The jury is still way out on APeX. Perhaps the reduction in blood flow to my tumor is just coincidence. Or maybe it was the result of my belief in the effectiveness of the Solution. There's no doubt that when hopes are raised the immune system responds. "Sure," Mark would say, "the placebo effect." Then again, *maybe*, against all odds, the APeX Solution will prove to be the gold in the 1% mine.

A SUMMING UP

So what have I learned that I can carry with me? How have I profited from my quest for the Enchanged Shotgun?

I see that the word "faith" occurs only once in this chapter. Yet from what I have observed, faith is one of the fundamental ingredients in the treatment choices we make. Many of the cancer survivors I've interviewed have supplemented traditional treatment with alternative therapies. And two things all these men have in common are faith in their chosen treatments, and hope. *Faith begets hope. Hope enables belief. Belief empowers healing.*

THE DOCTOR'S VIEW

Typical doctors' offices can be sterile, clinical, unfeeling, rushed and impersonal, and often increase anxiety rather than reduce it. Cancer patients lay their lives on the line when they consult a medical expert. How can they help but wonder, "Is it wise to trust someone who is unwilling to form an emotional attachment with his patients?"

As a rule, practitioners of complementary medicine seem far more willing to engage their human side, building hope and confidence in their patients. Their therapies help mitigate the stress and fear that increase cortisone levels in the blood, inhibiting the immune system. Benign treatments, delivered in an environment of hope and optimism, by reducing stress hormones that cripple immune function, can benefit patients in unexpected ways.

The placebo effect, though never fully understood or explained, is a real effect. It's power to help and comfort needy people should not be discounted.

4.

COMMUTING THE DEATH SENTENCE

Half our mistakes in life arise from feeling when we ought to think, and thinking when we ought to feel.

—JOHN CHURTON COLLINS

The best way I know to counter the fear that a diagnosis of prostate cancer means curtains is good information. You might think of this chapter as an orientation lecture from Prostate Cancer 101.

INTRODUCING THE PROSTATE GLAND

When we speak of the prostate *gland,* what are we really talking about? Glands are small, efficient factories. Glands make and secrete different substances such as mucus, sperm, earwax, various hormones, saliva and tears. Most glands simply drip their product into the bloodstream or into the channels that drain the gland. The prostate, however, has a strong capsule and a muscular structure surrounding it to compress and then fire its product, the sperm, at the intended target—an unfertilized egg.

The sperm—the wriggling packages of genetic material—make up only a small part of the white creamy matter called semen or the ejaculate. Most of the ejaculate is a manufactured product of the prostate itself, the fluid the sperm lives and swims in, and the fuel that provides the energy the sperm requires as it begins its journey in search of life's ultimate prize.

We learned in medical school that there are three major organs tightly packed into the narrow, bony pelvic region. We are all familiar with the bladder and the rectum, and the services they perform. But for some reason the golf-ball-size prostate gets no respect, as Rodney Dangerfield might say, until, with the onset of age, it swells, presses into the bladder and gets you up three times every night to urinate. Or becomes infected. Or harbors cancer.

WHAT IS CANCER?

Cancer consists of microscopic cells that don't know how to stop growing. When the multiplying cells attain a certain detectable size, they become a tumor. At some point during this developmental process, cancer cells break free from the mass, enter the bloodstream and land in another part of the body where they take root and form a new colony. This type of migration is called *metastasis*, from the Greek, "change of state." Once this process is set in motion, the new colonies spawn other colonies. Multiplication of new cells, new colonies and new tumors is now accelerating at a geometric rate. Sadly, the end of this story comes when there are so many tumors in so many vital sites—brain, liver, lung, kidneys—that organ failure and death occur.

PROSTATE CANCER IS NOT WHAT YOU THINK

Prostate cancer is incredibly common. Autopsies reveal that more than 50% of older men have it, live with it and die of something else, usually without ever even knowing they had it. Studies show that approximately 30% of fifty-year-old men and as many as 70% of eighty-year-old men harbor microscopic amounts of the disease.[1] In the opinion of one well-known urologist, "If you are over seventy, and you *don't* have prostate cancer, chances are you're a woman."

When I first see them, almost all my patients regard the diagnosis of any cancer as a death sentence. And yet prostate cancer is unique among cancers because the mortality rate is so low. Despite the fact that so many men have it, less than 3% of men in the U.S. die from it, and the mortality rate is dropping every year. A recent study, published in the *Journal of Clinical Oncology*, reported this remarkable statistic: *100%* of men with *Low-Risk* or *Intermediate-Risk* prostate cancer live more than ten years after diagnosis.[2] Clearly, there is an amazing divergence between the number of men who *have* prostate cancer and the number who *die* from it.

To better understand the surprisingly low malignant potential of prostate cancer, take the example of what is generally considered a worst-case scenario: a relapse after surgery or radiation. With most cancers, recurrence means imminent death, with survival times measured in months as shown in Table 1. However, read the bottom line of the table. The life expectancy for men with *recurrent* prostate cancer stretches out well past a decade. And remember that these statistics come from data collected on men who relapsed back in the 1990s. Men who relapse today will benefit from the discovery of many new medical advances over the next ten to fifteen years.

Table 1: The Uniqueness of Prostate Cancer

Cancer Type	Life Expectancy after Relapse from Surgery
Pancreatic	4 months
Kidney	6 months
Stomach	8 months
Lung	1 year
Colon	2 years
Breast	3 years
Prostate	**13 years**

Clearly, prostate cancer, *even the more serious relapsed form*, is nothing akin to an immediate death sentence.

FIVE FAVORABLE CHARACTERISTICS OF PROSTATE CANCER AND ITS TREATMENT

How can this cancer be so different from all the other cancers? Prostate cancer has five distinctive characteristics which, if taken together, provide a radically improved outlook for survival and cure.

The first characteristic is the *slow speed* of cancer growth. Cancers grow by doubling. Two becomes four. Four becomes eight . . . Experts estimate that about forty doublings are needed to reach the point where normal bodily functions are irrevocably impaired and death occurs. However, prostate cancer has been described as the "tortoise of cancers" because it replicates so slowly. Most other cancers have doubling times measured in weeks. Prostate cancer doubling times are measured in months or years.

The second characteristic is *the way prostate cancer spreads*. All malignancies can spread, or metastasize, wreaking havoc and impairing organ function. However, prostate cancer is unlike other common cancers such as lung or colon cancer, which metastasize indiscriminately to vital organs like the brain, lungs and liver. For reasons that remain unclear, the spread of prostate cancer is almost always restricted to two locations in the body: lymph nodes and bone marrow. Fortunately, these areas can tolerate the presence of cancer cells without malfunction.

The third characteristic of prostate cancer is *how easily it can be diagnosed at an early stage.* Because the prostate gland is no bigger than a walnut, its small size lends itself to accurate random needle sampling. Even tiny cancers are easily located by extracting tissue cores from the gland with a biopsy. Figure 1 indicates how difficult missing small cancers can be as the multiple biopsy cores are spaced evenly across the gland. In fact, biopsies are so effective that over-diagnosis is a real concern (see chapter 8).

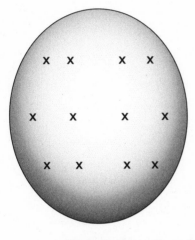

A two-centimeter (slightly less than one inch) hollow needle is inserted through the rectal wall and into the prostate at the locations marked with an **x**. A one-millimeter in diameter core of prostate tissue is thus removed from each location, systematically sampling the whole gland. Usually 12 to 18 cores are removed, depending on the size of the prostate gland.

Figure 1. Illustration of Needle Biopsy Sampling

The fourth favorable aspect of prostate cancer is an *early warning system called Prostate-Specific Antigen,* commonly known as PSA. Approved by the FDA in 1987, PSA is the mainstay for early diagnosis. Now, an additional test called PCA-3 is also available (see chapter 8). Prostate cancer is the only type of cancer with such powerful tests for detecting early stage disease.

The fifth favorable characteristic is the availability of *startlingly effective treatment.* For example, in the era before penicillin, in the time of our grandparents, the emotional reactions to the diagnosis of pneumonia or cancer were identical: both were equally deadly. Now that we have penicillin, pneumonia is hardly regarded as dangerous, let alone as serious as cancer. But what people fail to realize is that prostate cancer has its own "penicillin," drugs that work by blocking the production and activity of testosterone. Testosterone fuels prostate cancer growth, and blocking testosterone causes the disease to shrivel and regress. Prostate cancer is the *only* type of cancer susceptible to testosterone-inactivating pharmaceuticals. This important topic is addressed in detail in chapter 10.

THINGS YOUR UROLOGIST (AKA SURGEON) MAY NEGLECT TO TELL YOU

You may be thinking, "What about my Uncle Max who died of prostate cancer? If prostate cancer is so slow growing and so easy to diagnose, how come 27,000 men in the United States still die of it every year? What's going on?"

To counter inaccurate beliefs that are so widespread, this book addresses the great majority of men who do not have the life-threatening form of the disease, the 170,000 or so men diagnosed with prostate cancer annually who will live a normal life span. However, there remains a much smaller group of men who have a different type of prostate cancer, *High-Risk* disease, which, over a number of years, can evolve into a life-threatening situation.

The great peril is the misperception that prostate cancer is ONE illness. Dr. Anthony D'Amico, Chief of Radiation Therapy at Harvard Medical School, was the first to outline the three major categories or types of prostate cancer: *Low-*, *Intermediate-* and *High-Risk*.[3] His typing system is far more accurate than older staging systems and has become widely accepted as the industry standard. Therefore, because prostate cancer is not one illness, intelligent discussion about treatment can only begin after identifying the type. In the most simplistic terms, men with favorable types of prostate cancer should get either mild treatment or no treatment. Men with aggressive types should get aggressive treatment.

THE RISKS OF A PROSTATECTOMY MAY BE GREATER THAN THE THREAT OF THE DISEASE

Unfortunately, most patients and doctors alike either don't know or won't believe that anything called "cancer" deserves less than total eradication.

They also minimize or are unaware of the long-term implications of surgery. Certainly surgery or any of the other treatments discussed in this book should be considered for men with the more dangerous types of disease. However, considering that so many men these days are diagnosed with the *Low-Risk* variant, there needs to be some real soul searching before embarking on radical surgery for a condition that is not life threatening.

If prostate surgery were a simple procedure, say like an appendectomy, it could be recommended even if it failed to work in every case. When newly diagnosed patients converse with urologists, they often come away with the impression that prostate cancer surgery is fairly straightforward. In my experience, this impression is usually created by the less skillful surgeons. The most expert surgeons give lengthy descriptions of the challenging aspects of this complex and demanding operation.

The unpleasant fact is that any type of surgery brings with it the risk of infection, unremitting lifelong pain and temporary or permanent memory loss from anesthesia. Blood clots and heart attacks can also occur. These risks are not high in carefully selected individuals. But evidence indicates that many doctors fail to practice sufficient discrimination in selecting patients for surgical procedures, often, for example, electing to operate on men over age 70.[4]

Anatomically, the prostate is located in absolutely the wrong place for a simple surgical solution. Buried as it is, deep in the bony pelvis, access to the gland is extremely difficult, and considerable surgical difficulties have to be surmounted merely to arrive in its vicinity. Removing the gland itself is even more challenging.

The prostate is located within millimeters of the urinary bladder and the rectum, so there is zero tolerance for a slip of the scalpel. To make matters worse, there is a prolific venous blood supply surrounding the gland. Even the best surgeons can end up operating in a pool of blood, without a clear view of the object they are trying delicately to remove. Bleeding is often so prolific that some surgeons bank blood for transfusions during surgery. Yet the greatest danger from pooling blood in the operative field is the surgeon's restricted ability to see clearly in order to spare the minuscule nerves that control erections—nerves thinner than a human hair and invisible to the unaided eye. Some surgeons use microsurgery spectacles to improve their vision. With such an intricate and complex procedure, the 50% impotence rates reported by the best surgeons are hardly surprising.[5]

VERY UNPLEASANT CONSEQUENCES
AKA "COLLATERAL DAMAGE"

Even men who recover their erections after surgery undergo a protracted period of impotence, often lasting up to a year or more. During this time of enforced abstinence, as with any unused muscle, atrophy of the penis occurs. This means that of the men who end up recovering some degree of erectile function, *only 5% report that their erections are as good as before surgery.*[6] Additionally, despite claims from urologists who maintained for years that patients' complaints of penis shrinkage were anatomically impossible, diligent researchers have finally collected the necessary measurements. Unfortunately the studies show that shrinkage is common. The average amount is about one-half inch, although some men undergo considerably greater shrinkage.[7]

Another problem with surgery is the formation of scar tissue in the urethra, the passage from the bladder to the penis. The suture site where the severed urethra is reconnected can become constricted by scar tissue that blocks the flow of urine.[8] This may be correctable with urethral dilation, a process of forcing oversized, stainless steel probes up the penis to stretch out the ring of rock-hard tissue. Unfortunately, scar tissue is notoriously uncooperative, often refusing to stretch at all. In some cases the stretching fractures the brittle ring of tissue, resulting in permanent incontinence. If that happens, another operation is required to implant an artificial sphincter.

Urinary leakage is common even without stricture problems. The best urologists report that about 7% of their patients are left with permanent and constant urinary drainage.[9] Less-skilled surgeons have much higher rates. After surgery, most men experience some leakage whenever they cough, lift, bend over or simply laugh.[10]

There is another unfortunate and little publicized side effect of radical prostatectomy: interruption of the nerves that control rectal function. This condition can lead to irreversible loss of sphincter control, with unpleasant consequences such as fecal incontinence, otherwise known as "wet farts."[11]

THE MATTER OF QUALITY CONTROL

Levels of ability vary widely from surgeon to surgeon. So much skill is required to successfully perform a radical prostatectomy that being operated on by less than the very finest surgeon dramatically increases the chances for a poor outcome. In 2004, Dr. Peter Scardino, Chief of Urology at Memorial Sloan-Kettering, published a study documenting the differences in "talent" in this unregulated field. Scardino's study evaluated the surgical skill of twenty-six urologists on staff at Sloan-Kettering and Baylor. The indicator used to measure skill was the frequency of leaving cancer behind after the operation (the technical term is "a positive surgical margin"). The study reported that the best doctor in the group left cancer behind in 10% of his cases. The positive margin rates of the other twenty-five urologists ranged from 11 to 48%! These are disturbing statistics coming from two of the most prestigious university centers in the world.[12]

REFLECTIONS ON THE CURE RATE WITH SURGERY

What is the payoff for undergoing surgery? The best study addressing this question is a ten-year trial of almost 700 men performed in Scandinavia. The men volunteered to either undergo immediate surgery or to receive no treatment at all, depending on a coin flip. The results of the study were first published in the *New England Journal of Medicine* in May of 2005.[13] The survival rate with surgery was marginally better, but the differences between the two groups were surprisingly small. At the end of ten years, 10% of the men treated with surgery had died of prostate cancer. Among the men receiving no treatment whatsoever, 15% died. *The difference between the two groups was only 5%!* In other words, at best, only one out of every twenty men undergoing this difficult complex surgery actually had their lives extended.

ROBOTICS

No doubt you have heard these selling points for robotic surgery: less bloody, does less damage, you go home from the hospital in only one day and you'll be teeing off in a week. The recent infatuation with "the robot that can operate" would lead one to believe that extensive studies have shown superior results compared to the traditional get-in-there-and-get-blood-on-your-gloves approach. Despite the excitement and publicity, all the studies to date show that *the rates of incontinence and impotence with robotic surgery are identical to the results obtained with the traditional methods.*[14] One study comparing the two approaches shows more regret and dissatisfaction with robotic surgery, perhaps due to the unrealistically high expectations generated by enthusiastic surgeons.[15] Of equal concern are studies showing that urologists learning the new robotic technique require up to 250 practice procedures before their results are as good as those they achieve with the traditional method.

Make no mistake about it: a number of men who have surgery recover completely. These men often become zealous advocates for radical prostatectomy. They assume that others will sail through the operation just like they did. Other men, even though they have complications, put on a happy face, minimizing the daunting impact of impotence and incontinence. Men who want a realistic idea of what it is like to undergo surgery need to read Michael Korda's story in his book titled *Man to Man: Surviving Prostate Cancer*. Korda, then a senior editor at Simon & Schuster, vividly recounts his firsthand experience of a radical prostatectomy. What is eye opening is that his operation was done at Johns Hopkins by Patrick Walsh, the most famous and highly esteemed urologist in the world. Korda's experience with surgery was rather traumatic. Moreover, with the passage of time, it became apparent to him that the results of the procedure were considerably less satisfactory than he had anticipated.

GETTING THE APPROPRIATE MESSAGE ACROSS

As a prostate cancer specialist, I find that men are way too motivated to submit to radical treatment for what is typically a non–life-threatening condition. Despite quality research to the contrary, everyone finds it hard to believe that anything called cancer will stay dormant for years, even decades. In my opinion, men with the *Low-Risk* type of disease are surrendering to irrational and unwarranted fears. They are engaging in a costly overindulgence of their natural desire for closure, "to be rid of the cancer." Their real concern should be guarding and preserving quality of life. The number one priority should be avoiding side effects from unnecessary radical treatment.

THE PATIENT'S VIEW

If I had had this information when I began my own research, I would have been saved time, anguish and wasted effort. Truly I felt blessed when I was delivered into Mark's capable hands after it became apparent that I did have cancer. He listened to my concerns, gave me the information I needed, consulted with both Jeanne and me, and was willing to support me in my desire to wait and think about what I should do. I could have been one of these badly butchered men, had I fallen into another prostate camp.

The men to whom I showed this chapter all felt that it would have made their task far less daunting, if only by helping them identify the questions they needed to address. "Commuting the Death Sentence" provides a valuable ordnance map of the medical minefield.

5.

A BAND OF BROTHERS

What's in your mind is often quite literally or anatomically what is in
your body . . . What you have to understand is that there is a biology
of the individual as well as a biology of the disease, each affecting the
other. On the day of diagnosis we don't know either well enough to use
a pathology report to predict the future.

—BERNIE S. SIEGEL, MD

In the spring of 2001, two years after my second biopsy, a sudden jump
in my PSA from 7.4 to 20.3 sent me right up the wall. All my reasonable
assumptions shattered like glass and I suffered a full-blown panic attack.
The pressure to get treatment was immediate. PSA levels this high usually
indicate that the cancer has moved outside the prostate gland. If that was
the case, active surveillance was definitely no longer an option and neither
was surgery if the cancer had spread. My doctor on Maui urged me to
consider radiation. It was decision time.

The trouble was, I didn't feel up to making a decision of that magnitude. I had been feeling lousy—headachy, body aches, running a low
fever. At that point, my Refusenik self stepped in and decided for me:
Okay, so you'll probably have to do something, but there's no hurry.

It was a Saturday, the day the big outrigger canoes would be putting
to sea. Why not go paddling? I grabbed my paddle and drove to the Wailuku harbor. The sun was shining; a breeze was kicking up tiny whitecaps.
Down on the sand, the last outrigger canoe was just loading up, and they
were short a man.

When you're in only mediocre physical condition, and everyone else
in the boat is thirty-five years younger than you, there's no energy to spend
on the state of your prostate. You row. You sweat, you ache and you pull
your paddle. We were out near the breakwater when the coxswain gave
the order to stop paddling. I was resting on my paddle, getting my breath

and watching a giant cruise ship drop anchor across the bay, when I had an idea: I still felt really crappy with these flu-like symptoms, and it occurred to me that my elevated PSA just might be caused by an infection of some sort.

As soon as we came ashore and beached the canoe, I drove to see my family doctor, Joel Friedman, upcountry in Kula. I told him my theory, got a prescription and began treating myself with a course of the antibiotic Cipro (Ciprofloxacin). After ten days I felt much better and, more to the point, my PSA had dropped back to 9.25—far from perfect, but a big improvement. I was pleased with myself. I was trusting my instincts, taking responsibility for my health. I was never quite sure what the term "proactive" meant, but I figured it's what I was being.

Joel was still concerned, so he sent me to Maui Memorial for a bone scan. Much to my relief, there was no sign of metastasis. However, Jeanne was not entirely reassured, and she convinced me that I should see John Kurhanewicz, PhD, at the Magnetic Resonance Science Center in San Francisco to make sure the cancer had not spread outside the gland. So at the beginning of June, I flew to San Francisco for a spectrographic endorectal MRI. The result was mixed. There was no evidence of "extracapsular extension," meaning the cancer was still confined within the prostate, but the tumor was growing. Not fast, but growing.

A BAND OF BROTHERS

After my anxiety over my skyrocketing PSA, I suddenly felt a howling need for the company of other men who had been through what I was going through. I needed to find a prostate cancer support group. My friend David Derris told me about a monthly meeting that was held in Conference Room #1 at Kaiser Permanente's Wailuku Clinic. This was my first support group, so it wasn't until I later attended other groups on the mainland that I realized how quirky the Kaiser group was, and learned that all support groups are not created equal.

First of all, the older guys didn't like coming out at night. But what they didn't like even more was the idea that they needed to change their eating habits. There was one upcountry farmer named Pedro, who was seventy-three, overweight and diabetic. He wasn't a suitable candidate for surgery because of his health, so his doctor had recommended radiation, and his wife did her best to provide him with a better diet. Only there was no way

Pedro was going to give up gorging on Portuguese sausages and the heavily sugared donuts called *malasadas*. In spite of the radiation, he had a recurrence in a matter of months.

Another drawback with the Kaiser group was the absence of an experienced moderator to help with intimacy questions, particularly since the meetings were attended by a number of wives. When it came to "talking story," there was never any mention of what is, for most men, the big issue: sexual dysfunction. If I brought up the subject, I got, "Oh yeah, everything's fine. It's all *pau*" (Hawaiian for "okay"). But you could see from the faces of the wives that it was far from *pau*. And yet when a talented husband and wife team, John and Natalie Tyler, psychologists specializing in couples' problems, visited the support group and offered their help, the men were just too uncomfortable to discuss anything to do with sexual intimacy. The Tylers got no takers from among Maui's prostate cancer population. Couples therapy? Talk about your sex life? Forget it. For those guys, "denial" was definitely not a river in Egypt. Eventually the Kaiser support group just shut down.

Finding the right support group is one of the best things you can do for yourself following a diagnosis of prostate cancer. Since leaving Maui, I have participated in groups in Los Angeles, Santa Fe, New York and London. In the best groups, men share their stories and offer one another valuable advice from their own experience. At times they are even willing to discuss the emotionally painful stuff: their loss of libido, the embarrassment of growing breasts, their fear of never having another erection. But that kind of openness is the exception rather than the rule and varies widely from group to group, meeting to meeting. Still, you are likely to learn more about coping with the emotional side of this disease from men who have actually been through surgery, radiation, cryotherapy or hormone blockade than you will learn from your urologist who, chances are, hasn't had prostate cancer. What's more, your local support group is often your best resource for referrals, for learning the names of the most experienced (and best liked) prostate specialists in your area. And as Mark never tires of reminding his patients, "Finding the right doctor is just as important as finding the right treatment."

In most states, you will find active prostate cancer groups that provide treatment advice and emotional support. Organizations such as Us TOO, the American Cancer Society's Man to Man, and Malecare have Web sites that offer valuable guidance and provide the names and locations of meetings in your area. Other excellent resources include Michael Milken's Prostate Cancer Foundation (PCF) and the Prostate Cancer Research Institute (PCRI) where you will find a number to call at any time to speak with a Helpline Advisor.* And when in doubt, there's always "Dr. Google" for referrals.

THE PROSTATE CANCER CAREGIVERS HALL OF FAME

Sometimes the volunteer leaders of support groups are men who, while waging their own battles against prostate cancer, are generous in sharing their experience and knowledge with men just beginning the journey. These seasoned veterans are not medically trained or licensed, yet they are wise in the ways of the disease and free of any bias. They are caregivers in the best sense.

Since my diagnosis, I have developed many prostate cancer friendships, close connections with very special men I never would have met without the disease. For two years, I was blessed to have such a relationship with Bill Blair. I was able to call Bill any time, day or night, and tell him what I was going through, especially when I lost my nerve. Bill was a peerless friend and resource: he knew the medicine, he had a ton of experience and he had a great heart. With him, as the song says, "the telephone line was a lifeline."

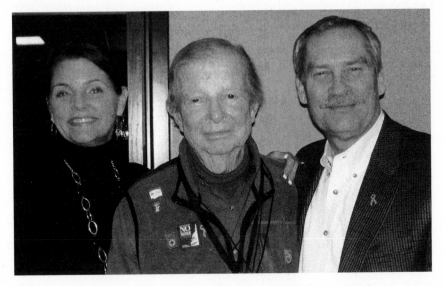

Bill Blair (center) with Terri Gibbons and Tom Kirk of Us TOO.

* How to contact these and other support organizations will be found at the back of the book under "Web Sites."

This photograph of Bill was taken in 2008 when he received the Ed Kaps Hope Award from Terri Gibbons and Tom Kirk. I keep it taped to the shelf above my desk, so I can see Bill every time I look up from my computer.

I came to appreciate Bill's indomitable spirit as he fought with his very advanced disease. Sometimes when I called him he was laboring to breathe, assisted by an oxygen tank. But he always took my call and was always ready to listen and talk. There were days when I thought he was nearing the end, but then he soldiered back. The last time we spoke, Bill was in the hospital, in intensive care. But even there, right by his bed, was the phone. On his last day, with a breathing apparatus and a clamp over one finger to measure blood oxygen, he asked June, his wife, to find him a pad of paper and a pencil.

"He was recording data," June explained, "even as he was dying." Then she hesitated a moment before adding softly, "He believed he still had a future."

Well, that's the truth. Bill does still have a future: it resides in the hearts and minds of all of us whom he befriended and guided and loved. He's gone now, but when the lab calls and tells me, "Your PSA has dropped from 4.9 to 3.8," I think, *See, Bill, I'm doing great!* When I call my English filmmaker pal, Harvey Frost, and hear how he's riding out his bone metastases, I tell Bill, *Ain't Harvey a lamp in the darkness!* Bill continues to make a difference in the lives of all of us who knew him. He lives in our shared memories, our bursts of renewed courage, our wild life-giving laughter.

THE WOMEN WHO LOVE US

Men are conditioned not to whine or complain. Although we are prepared to speak openly in support groups about our treatment, we don't readily share our experience of sensitive issues, or how we cope with the emotional consequences of prostate cancer treatments. So thank God for the women! Over and over, I have been touched by their willingness to share their feelings and face the issues that really matter.

I remember one woman telling a group how, when her husband was seriously depressed about having to wear diapers after a radical prostatectomy, she would struggle to remain upbeat and positive around him. Then she would break down and weep when she was alone. Another woman confessed that when her husband lost his libido and his ability to have erections, he closed off emotionally, totally shut her out. "But for me," she said, "sex is not *just* about erections. What I want most is *emotional* closeness, and I need to be touched, cuddled, held. I need my man to find other ways of expressing love and being intimate."

However, not many women are bold enough to bring up these sensitive matters in a men's support group. And there are very few experts who have looked into the psychological and emotional dynamics of the spouses of men with prostate cancer. Canadian psychologist Dr. Sylvie Aubin, PhD, at the Seattle Cancer Care Alliance of the Fred Hutchinson Cancer Research Center, is one of those few. She ran a unique women's support group that focused on the psychosocial issues that impact both men *and* their spouses following a diagnosis of prostate cancer.

When I asked Dr. Aubin to share with me her observations regarding the women, she told me they are only able to talk about their sadness, their fear, the possibility of "life without him" when they are in the group. At home, they always need to be brave, to contain their emotions, to become — like their men — solution oriented.

"Men's support groups are very focused on treatment," Dr. Aubin told me. "Actually, men prefer to listen to a lecturer. My women's group is about the experience and the challenges. Men aren't comfortable looking at or dealing with intimacy issues. They're socialized to 'fix the broken chair.' It's very hard to get men to open up about how they feel. And the stigmatization is heavy. They think that if they talk about their emotions people will think, 'Oh, so he probably can't perform'."

Dr. Aubin was emphatic about how important women are as providers of accurate information, especially when it comes to a man's emotional state. "We ask, 'Have you been feeling sad or depressed?' and he goes, 'No, not at all.' Then we ask the spouse, and she says, 'Yes, he's depressed all the time.' Doctors, by and large, focus only on the technical aspects of treatment. Rarely is a man going to feel comfortable bringing up his emotional problems in a medical setting. However, a lot of women are also reluctant to talk openly about their intimate lives, which is why groups like mine, that create a safe place for women to talk about *their* sensitive issues, are few and far between."

It took a while but I finally began to appreciate the extraordinary role women play in our lives when we are diagnosed. It is often the women who buy and read the books, study the medical literature, do research on the Internet, locate the best doctors in their area, ask all the questions and insist on second opinions. It is the women who help us with the hard treatment choices, make sure we keep our appointments and remind us to take our medications. They become our nurses and our cheerleaders, our live-in therapists when we become fearful or depressed. Jeanne has been my rock during all the years I have spent in the prostate cancer minefield.

THE TYRANNY OF STATISTICS

Among the many things I learned in the support groups I attended is that every man's prostate cancer is different, as is his general health, his diet, his lifestyle and his mindset. You need to make sure that all of these elements are taken into account before you decide on a treatment—or on no treatment. I have met with men who had been railroaded into questionable therapies, scared half to death over nonthreatening cancers and robbed of free choice by a system that is spinning out of control. And I have met far too many men who were told they were going to die, based on a pathology report and a fistful of statistics.

When you are first diagnosed, you will often be provided with literature filled with numerical tables, statistics and graphs that are both overwhelming and scary as hell. Your response to them is critical. *Statistics measure populations; they don't apply to individuals.* But if you allow them to frighten and depress you, they become the stuff of self-fulfilling prophecy.

One fellow I got to know, Sam Guffy, a southerner who spoke in a drawl, talked about "statistical *ovuh*load." At the time of his diagnosis, he was told he had a 23% chance the cancer was still contained in the gland, a 57% chance it had penetrated the prostate wall, a 10% chance of seminal vesicle involvement and a 9% chance the cancer had spread to the lymph nodes. "Well, *shee-it!*" he said, "Try sorting out that lot! And anyway, I'm not a damned statistic, I'm a *person!*" I told him the Mark Twain quip about the three varieties of dishonesty, each worse than the one before: "lies, damned lies and statistics."

Sam Guffy is right. Statistics and pathology reports tell only part of the story. What's missing is the influence exerted by all the variables and intangibles that, as Sam would say, make you a person.

INTANGIBLE FACTORS

There are actually studies showing that men who attend support groups live longer than those who don't. Speculation as to why this might be the case usually centers on mind–body interactions.

Sir Max Beerbohm, the British humorist, once began a radio broadcast with this disclaimer: "Ladies and gentlemen, I'm afraid my subject is rather an exciting one and as I don't like excitement, I shall approach it in a gentle, timid, roundabout way." Well, my subject is an exciting one, but I intend to plunge right in. It concerns the healing power of mind–body communication and the intangible factors that I am convinced have strengthened me on this long prostate cancer journey.

Among these intangibles I include a positive attitude, tranquility of mind, a shared responsibility for my own healing, an independent and contrary spirit and large doses of hope, faith, belief and gratitude. Throw in a willingness and ability to express my needs and emotions, an irreverent sense of humor and both a strong will to live and reasons to look forward to each day and to the future.

Largely thanks to the groundbreaking work of Candace Pert, PhD, and leading medical innovators like Carl Simonton, Bernie Siegel, Larry Dossey and Andrew Weil, there is growing acceptance of the idea that what we believe, what we think and what we feel manifests in our bodies. And yet as far as I am aware, no one in the scientific community has assembled data on the presence of these intangibles in a population sample made up from the thousands of people who continue to do well despite a dismal prognosis, or on those who were given a death sentence and who are still alive years later. I count myself as part of that latter group.

So what's the problem here? Funding? Skepticism? The magnitude of the challenge? From a statistician's point of view, these intangibles are qualitatively elusive, difficult to measure and lack a convenient scale of quantitative distribution. However, there is already a significant body of anecdotal evidence that testifies to the role intangible factors play in the course of any serious illness. This is hardly a new idea. It was Hippocrates, the father of Western medicine, who declared that he would rather know what sort of person has a disease than what sort of disease a person has.

ENTER THE REMARKABLE BRUCE LIPTON

One more voice needs to be heard on the issue of mind–body medicine, that of cellular biologist Bruce Lipton, PhD, author of *The Biology of Belief: Unleashing the Power of Consciousness, Matter and Miracles.* Lipton believes that all the tools to heal us are built into our biology, and that it's only because, in our society, we have been programmed to be dependent entirely on doctors, that we have forgotten or abandoned this innate ability. For some time now, genetic triggering has been the flavor of the month, the theory being that our genes turn the cells on and off, thereby affecting cancer growth or absence thereof. For decades, Lipton has been saying that it is the *micro-environment* that activates or suppresses the genes. And what produces the "climate" in the micro-environment? Things like emotional state, level of anxiety, the effect of stress hormones and all those other intangible factors. Since this regulatory system is above or superior to the actual genes, the scientific name for this field is "epigenetics."

According to Lipton, individuals with similar or identical genes will progress differently with, say, prostate cancer, because what happens to each of them is determined less by their genetic predisposition than by the weather conditions in their micro-environments.

I am only mentioning Lipton's work in passing, but I encourage you to find out when he will be lecturing in your area, and go! Lipton's second home is on stage, in front of an audience. He'll be good for whatever ails you.

WHAT IS IT YOU CAN'T HAVE WITHOUT A PROSTATE?

If you guessed an erection, you were on the right path. But for Jeanne and me, the answer was a baby. Despite my age, we were still hoping to have a child. I had never informed myself about the way things work regarding insemination. In simple terms, it goes something like this: the sperm is carried by a continuous structure of hollow tubes from the testes to the epididymus to the vas deferens (in doc-speak "the vas") to the seminal vesicles, where it is stored, matures and then gets introduced through the ejaculatory ducts into the prostatic urethra where it's mixed with prostatic fluid. The approximate recipe calls for ½ cc of sperm to 4½ cc of prostatic fluid; mix well, and you've got the ejaculate. Then comes the fun part. And hopefully, in the fullness of time, the baby.

If, however, you have prostate cancer, and you want to hedge your bets, there's another option: you can always bank your sperm and put your trust in artificial insemination. During our time on Maui, Jeanne and I looked into that possibility. I even went to a clinic in Honolulu and made a deposit. However, the experience of banking my sperm was not too cool.

First of all, I learned that it's prudent to store about five vials of ejaculate, meaning that in my case, I'd have to fly five different times from Maui to Honolulu, then pay five monthly storage charges. Not that I was unwilling to lay out the money. But five sessions alone in a tiny room with a stack of grotty boob-and-beaver magazines and my reluctant imagination was the total opposite of a turn-on.

Even more depressing, when I had my sperm checked out, I learned that it was affected by "low motility," as in sluggish. Not a good sign. You want sperm that, if not sprinting, can at least jog. Add to that a low total sperm count and a less than reassuring number of so-called normal forms and the odds of having a baby begin to resemble those of being struck by lightning.

I made only two deposits and then decided to hang on to my prostate and treat it respectfully for as long as I safely could. I never returned to withdraw my deposits.

STRATEGIC ALLIANCES

It's a good thing to hold your ground in the face of pressure from authority figures who ride roughshod over your sense of your own best interests. It is, I suggest, even more important to join forces with physicians you can trust to support you in the decisions that *you* feel are right for you. It was my good fortune to find two such physicians: Mark Scholz, a prostate oncologist, and Duke Bahn, an interventional radiologist and leading practitioner in the study and treatment of prostate cancer. Because of my history of gnarly interactions with urologists, my friend David Derris recommended that I fly to Los Angeles for a consultation with Dr. Scholz who, he explained, was one of a small number of oncologists whose singular focus is prostate cancer.

My first meeting with Mark took place in late June 2001. He had his lab do blood work and he reviewed my medical history. My PSA at that time had risen to 10.6, but as my recent tests had shown no bone metastases and no sign of the cancer having escaped the gland, Mark agreed to support me in my determination to avoid invasive and radical treatment and to abet me in continuing to pursue, for the time being, a policy of watchful waiting.

Over the coming year, Mark and I had several discussions about the widespread collateral damage caused by inappropriate or inexpert treatments and his commitment to reducing the number of unnecessary biopsies performed every year in the U.S. Then in July 2002, when my PSA climbed to 14.8, Mark sent me to Ventura to see Duke Bahn, one of a handful of radiologists who use color Doppler ultrasound to determine whether there is angiogenesis, or blood flow, to the tumor.

The news was not good. The ultrasound confirmed that, since the MRI the previous year, the tumor had continued to grow and that there was significant blood flow.

On receiving Dr. Bahn's results, Mark ordered a batch of tests to establish that the cancer had not spread, and we began to talk seriously about hormone blockade. But in typical Refusenik fashion, I continued to drag my feet. And my PSA continued to climb.

THE DOCTOR'S VIEW

Ralph does an excellent job of showing how dependent we are on others for good information and support. It may be the boldness of a spouse or companion who accompanies you to the doctor and is willing to ask pointed questions. And then, after the doctor visit is over, there is someone to help you remember what was said, someone who can discuss the merits of what is being recommended.

Networking in a support group is also valuable because the attendees have only two motives for being there: to be helped and to help others. It's not unusual to run across unique individuals who have dedicated countless hours to background research. These laymen can become so knowledgeable that the expertise of the average urologist pales by comparison. Spouses have opportunities to interact with other women who are dealing with similar issues. Last but not least, at a support group you can conveniently query a large number of people about the doctors in your community. How better to identify the good, the bad and the ugly than by talking to other consumers?

6.

INTRODUCING ACTIVE SURVEILLANCE

New ideas are always suspected, and usually opposed, without any other reason but because they are not already common.

—JOHN LOCKE

After men and their partners get beyond the initial shock of a prostate cancer diagnosis, they often ask me how their doctor could have been so biased toward a single treatment. After all, as a professional isn't he supposed to lay aside his own personal interests and adopt those of his patient? How can he counsel surgery or radiation when in fact the condition could be safely monitored?

There are various explanations. Physicians, as well as patients, struggle with the incongruity of simply watching cancer. When cancer is mentioned, everyone automatically assumes it's deadly. Currently, most doctors still adhere to the policy of treating everyone. Naturally, doctors tend to be nervous about new thinking or treatments. It's safer to stay within the familiar bounds of customary and traditional protocols. When treatment is outside the standard of care *and if something goes wrong* a lawsuit could follow. Lastly, we can't forget that there are financial issues at stake. When seeing a patient for the first time, some doctors may be thinking, "This man is so scared. There is no way he will be willing to forgo treatment. If I don't do the treatment, he will just go down the street and get it from my competitor." Unfortunately, this is a fact of life for doctors.

A PATIENT LEADS THE WAY

My introduction to active surveillance started way back in the mid-1990s when a successful, fifty-five-year-old movie actor whom I will call John came to me for his umpteenth opinion for newly diagnosed prostate cancer. He had what we today would term *Low-Risk* disease. At that time, most doctors, myself included, had hardly a notion of a "harmless" cancer. As would be expected, all his doctors recommended surgery. However, John was very concerned about losing sexual function. He even convinced one of his doctors to try what at that time was a very unorthodox approach, treatment with Casodex, a pill to block testosterone. This pill reduced his libido, so he stopped treatment after thirty days.

After John came to me, our idea was to try a much milder medication called Proscar. But even this was unacceptable to John. Ultimately, he simply changed his diet and refused to undergo any treatments at all. He did, however, continue careful monitoring. That was over thirteen years ago. To this day, John continues to be checked regularly with PSA blood tests, ultrasound and MRI scans, and an occasional repeat biopsy. He has never needed additional therapy and his PSA remains stable.

John's unwillingness to have treatment was mostly his doing. He gives me credit for supporting his decision but I argue that he didn't give me any choice. Certainly I was aware of studies from Europe documenting that untreated prostate cancer can remain stable for decades. But most of the men in those studies were twenty years older than John.

KEEPING AN OPEN MIND

Looking back over my career, I seem to be more comfortable with ambiguity than many of my peers. I get impatient with pat and simple answers. I think my restless nature was reinforced by five years at USC county hospital, a place where the unusual is commonplace and there is plenty of room for a maverick to roam. After USC, I became the oncology director of an HMO in Cerritos, California. I selected an HMO because I thought their culture of using the minimum (and the least expensive) form of treatment was similar to my philosophy. But I didn't realize how quickly medicine was changing. New and more effective drugs were coming on the market. As it turned out, I had misjudged my temperament. On repeated occasions I clashed with the HMO hierarchy about access to new drug and treatment options for my patients. Within two years I wanted a change.

I decided to enter private practice. From a financial point of view it seemed like a foolish decision. In the late 1980s, the growing HMOs were a powerful economic force. The future of private practice looked bleak. But I was getting worn down by the obligation of placing a dollar figure on every medical decision. Diagnosing and treating patients is challenging enough, even without the distorting influence of administrative pressures to minimize costs. Although a future in private practice seemed doubtful, I could not stomach the fact that after five years of undergraduate training, four years of medical school, and five more years of postgraduate fellowship training, my life would end up being spent watching pennies for an insurance company masquerading as a medical group.

EVERY PATIENT REQUIRES INDIVIDUALIZED CARE

I found a position in private practice with a medical oncologist working in the San Fernando Valley near Los Angeles. This is where I first started seeing men with earlier stage prostate cancer. I was initially surprised by my new partner's highly personalized treatment philosophy. He seemed totally unconcerned that his approach was different from that of other doctors. When I questioned him he stated flatly, "I treat patients the way I would treat myself or my family." This was a revolutionary statement compared to the impersonal scientific attitude encouraged in my medical training where decisions were reached by consensus, and being different raised questions about your judgment. Before long, however, I became convinced that his approach was superior. His patient-first philosophy was creative and personal, taking full advantage of new medical advances as soon as they came on the market.

PUTTING BELIEFS INTO ACTION

Shortly thereafter I had a chance to exercise this new approach with Walter Bates, a retired police officer who was consulting me because his PSA was rising after surgery. The problem for me was that medical oncology training programs only instruct in the management of *advanced* prostate cancer. Urologists are expected to handle all the early-stage disease. So, as preparation for our meeting I had to educate myself about a type of cancer known as *PSA-relapsed disease*. To start, I purchased a small 175-page book titled *Clinical Management of Prostate Cancer*.

To my surprise, in the whole book, prostate-specific antigen (PSA) was referenced only in two places! In the author's opinion, now laughable in retrospect (this was 1989), "PSA is unlikely to be useful as a screening test for segments of the population." His negative viewpoint about PSA was understandable as PSA testing had been FDA approved only two years previously and doctors had yet to gain familiarity with its use. The other reference in the book to PSA was relevant to Walter's case: "PSA has been shown to be a sensitive and specific marker for detection of recurrent disease after surgery."

So a detectable and rising PSA meant that cancer was still present somewhere in Walter's body; the surgery had failed to eradicate it. Walter underwent bone and body scans, which were clear, indicating that the recurrent cancer was probably microscopic, too small to be seen on the scans. Yet both of us were concerned that without treatment bone metastases were bound to eventually appear. Walter was impatient to do something. His attitude was, "Why should I wait until I have detectable chunks of cancer in my bones before I initiate therapy?"

RESISTANCE FROM DEFENDERS OF THE STATUS QUO

Walter's urologist was recommending that testosterone inactivating pharmaceuticals (TIP) be withheld until bone metastases were present. But the urologist's recommendation contradicted one of the cardinal principles of my medical oncology training: starting treatment at an earlier stage gives better long-term results. So Walter and I faced a dilemma: Should we submit to the prevailing belief espoused by surgeons, or follow the principles of treatment developed by experts through studies of other types of cancer? Walter ultimately decided to start TIP. Subsequently, over the next thirteen years, he underwent three one-year courses. In 2009 he was doing well; his PSA was undetectable.

In 2004, eight years after Walter and I first anguished about whether or not to start TIP, studies confirming superior outcomes for the early initiation of TIP prior to the onset of bone metastasis were published.[1] At the present time, the general practice is to start it immediately in men with higher Gleason scores or rapidly rising PSA levels. Leaving behind the old ways of doing things and embracing new thinking is challenging for all of us. I must confess that when studies advocating active surveillance started coming out, even though I had been monitoring John all those years, I was still unconvinced. True, John had done well. But was he just lucky? And to make things easier for me, John was taking most of the responsibility for the decision to forgo treatment. That's quite different from me as a physician *advocating* active surveillance.

JOHN WAS NOT THE ONLY ONE

Throughout the years there have been others who were reluctant to have radical therapy. Sam Slater, a young-at-heart guy who likes to drive race cars, was first diagnosed in 1998 at the age of sixty-one. His PSA was 5.8. Only one of his six biopsy cores contained Gleason 6 disease. When I recommended treatment he flatly refused. Throughout the years Sam has been monitored with periodic endorectal MRI and color Doppler ultrasound studies (chapter 14), which have been stable. His PSA continues to hover in the 4 to 5 range. In September 2007 a color Doppler ultrasound study detected a cancerous spot in the left base. The following year a repeat evaluation appeared to show slight enlargement of the spot. We have been recommending another biopsy, but after enjoying a great quality of life for so many years, Sam is understandably reluctant to intervene further.

Independent thinkers are the norm with my clientele. (Ralph, my co-author, certainly fits the bill!) Larry Simons is also among my forward-minded patients. He is an executive who was diagnosed with two cores of low-grade prostate cancer in March of 1996 at the age of sixty. At that time his PSA was 4.8. Throughout the years he has followed an active surveillance protocol with periodic endorectal MRI and color Doppler ultrasound scans. The tests have shown a slow enlargement of a small tumor in the apex of his gland. In October 2008, when Larry was seventy-two, his PSA had risen to 7 but the tumor was unchanged.

PROSTATE CANCER STATISTICS

Considering how well these men have fared, perhaps watching prostate cancer is not as crazy as it sounds. The overall statistics are convincing. For the last two decades, over 200,000 men have been diagnosed annually with prostate cancer. However, the death rate is only 27,000. So what happens to the 173,000 who don't die? Well, we know that over time 25,000 to 30,000 of them do develop metastatic disease. However, they die of other causes such as old age or heart disease. In other words, they die *with* but not *of* metastasis. That leaves 143,000 who never develop metastasis or die of the disease. Liberal use of surgery and radiation can't explain such high survival rates because studies show that surgery reduces mortality by 5% at most. So if we subtract another 5% of men who are cured by treatment, *that still leaves 135,000 men diagnosed every year who will live out a normal life expectancy and never suffer metastasis.*

Dr. Laurence Klotz, a visionary urologist from Toronto, runs the numbers slightly differently: "While the lifetime risk of *being diagnosed* with prostate cancer is one out of six, prior to the advent of PSA screening *the risk of death* from prostate cancer was only one out of forty. Despite this large discrepancy, 94% of men with *Low-Risk* disease are still receiving radical treatment. In the rare instances where a life is saved by surgery— thought to be about one out of a hundred in men with *Low-Risk* disease— *that man's 'early death' occurs an average of sixteen years after diagnosis and only four years prior to when death would be expected to occur from old age.* At best, surgery only extends average life expectancy by 1.2 months!"[2]

Dr. Klotz goes on to point out that with active surveillance, men still have plenty of opportunity for treatment. When men are watched closely, treatment can be started at the first sign of progression, while the disease is still curable. The fact that medical technology improves every year provides an even greater incentive for delaying treatment.

DEFINING A HARMLESS TYPE OF CANCER

Believe it or not, studies of *Low-Risk* prostate cancer patients actually show them to have better ten-year survival after diagnosis than men who have never been diagnosed with prostate cancer! This jarring truth is explained by the fact that "being diagnosed" means that you are in the medical system, that your blood pressure, cholesterol and other important health-related factors are being monitored.[3] The benefit of simply getting to a doctor and receiving routine medical care outweighs the minuscule disadvantage of being diagnosed with *Low-Risk* disease.

As we pointed out in chapter 4, prostate cancer is not a single disease. Rather it should be thought of as three distinct types: *Low-Risk,*

Intermediate-Risk and *High-Risk* (see Table 2). Most men are totally un-aware that *Low-Risk* disease is harmless. Instead, their diagnosis throws them into a panic. What they need to know is that embarking on active surveillance is not like playing a cancer lottery. Widely accepted methods based on Gleason grade, PSA and biopsy findings can determine who can be safely monitored and who is better off starting treatment immediately. Reputable studies show that the mortality of *Low-Risk* and *Intermediate-Risk* disease within the first ten years of diagnosis is negligible.[4]

Table 2: Determining Your Risk Status

Cancer Risk or "Type"	Gleason Score	% of Biopsy Cores with Cancer	PSA Level	PSA* Velocity	PSA** Density	Digital Rectal Exam
Low	< 7	< 34%	< 10	< 2	< 0.15	No Nodule
Intermediate	7	34–50%	10–20	< 2	> 0.15	Small Nodule
High	> 7	> 50%	> 20	> 2		Larger Nodule

* PSA Velocity = How many points the PSA goes up in the previous year
**PSA Density = PSA divided by the size of the prostate in cubic centimeters (cc)

A PROSPECTIVE STUDY OF ACTIVE SURVEILLANCE

Back in the mid 1990s Dr. Klotz set about proving the feasibility of active surveillance by recruiting 300 volunteers. Most of the men were *Low-Risk* though some were *Intermediate-Risk*. These men underwent PSA and dig-ital rectal exams quarterly. They had prostate biopsies performed one and three years after initial diagnosis. Treatment with surgery or radiation was administered only if their PSA rose excessively or if the findings on DRE or biopsy worsened.[2]

After five and a half years of observation, one-third of the men (101 men) had come off observation and undergone some form of treatment. The reasons for initiating treatment differed. Forty-five of those men (15%) came off surveillance because of a rising PSA level: nine men (3%) had changes in their digital rectal examination, twelve men (4%) showed worse findings on subsequent biopsy, and thirty-six (12%) decided to have some form of therapy even though their situation was stable. Two men with rapidly rising PSA levels died from prostate cancer despite treatment, but at the time of publication, no other men had developed metastatic disease.

EXPERT CONSENSUS

The results of this study, published in the *Journal of Clinical Oncology* in 2005, were not lost on one of the most eminent doctors in the United States, Dr. Peter Carroll, Chief of Urology at the University of California at San Francisco. In 2007 Dr. Carroll convened the first Conference on Active Surveillance for over 200 of the leading prostate cancer experts in the world. The conference attendees were asked to form a consensus on how to select men who would be eligible to embark on active surveillance. Parameters for selection were initially developed by a working group of about twenty physicians (of which I was one) and subsequently proposed to the whole body of the conference, where they were voted on and accepted.

The agreed-upon standards relied heavily on the published research of Dr. Jonathan Epstein from Johns Hopkins, who defined *Low-Risk* prostate cancer as a Gleason Grade less than 7, a PSA less than 10, and three or fewer biopsy cores positive for cancer. Age restrictions, an important component of the old approach of watchful waiting, were specifically rejected as unnecessary for embarking on active surveillance.* The conference attendees believed that if the basic requirements of *Low-Risk* disease are met, as shown in Table 2, *men at any age could safely undergo active surveillance*. As men get older (i.e., into their late seventies) the criteria can be liberalized, allowing men with higher risk disease to pursue active surveillance. As life expectancy diminishes, even aggressive cancers have insufficient time to cause harm. The ultimate goal of active surveillance is not forgoing treatment indefinitely. *The goal of active surveillance is selective treatment that is restricted only to those who really need it.* Close

---

* Watchful waiting was an approach used prior to the discovery of PSA. In years past it was known that prostate cancer was likely to grow slowly. Older men who had nodules detected on digital rectal examination were unlikely to have the disease progress within their expected lifetime. Therefore they were advised to forgo treatment and call for an appointment if their bones began to hurt. If that occurred, they were treated with surgical castration.

monitoring of the cancer's behavior in each individual is the best method for determining who needs treatment and who can safely continue being watched.

HOW DANGEROUS IS WAITING?

Of course the crucial question is, "How often, by delaying treatment, will we end up losing the chance for a cure?" Researchers from Johns Hopkins addressed this question by evaluating the stage of cancer found after surgery in men who had been on active surveillance for some time but later progressed and needed surgery. The researchers compared their surgical findings with another large group of men who had undergone immediate surgery. Reassuringly, the study found that the extent of disease in both groups was equivalent. The men who waited were no worse off than the men who had immediate treatment.[5]

WHAT DOES ACTIVE SURVEILLANCE REQUIRE?

How exactly is active surveillance carried out? Most centers rely on quarterly PSA testing and repeat biopsies. Johns Hopkins has the most aggressive program as they recommend a biopsy every year. At the 2007 Active Surveillance Conference, annual biopsies were thought to be excessive. The conference attendees recommended a biopsy after one year, subsequently repeating it every two to three years. At the center where I practice, we generally guide the decision to do a repeat biopsy on the basis of PSA, PCA-3 and prostate imaging with either color Doppler ultrasound or spectrographic endorectal MRI (Table 3).

Table 3: Active Surveillance Protocol

Baseline spectrographic endorectal MRI and color Doppler ultrasound
PSA every 3 months
PCA-3* at baseline and every 6–12 months
Rectal examination every 6 months
Color Doppler ultrasound semiannually
Spectrographic endorectal MRI annually

*PCA-3 is a urine test for diagnosing prostate cancer. We have also found it to be a useful ancillary test for monitoring men on active surveillance.

THE "SYSTEM" RESISTS CHANGE

As I have said, both patients and doctors struggle with the idea that anything called cancer can be safely observed. However, with *Low-Risk* prostate cancer, the evidence is mounting that active surveillance is both sensible and safe.[6,7,8,9] Unfortunately, despite accumulating evidence, many doctors are offering only lip service to the idea. Dr. Anthony Zeitman, a radiation therapist from Massachusetts General Hospital, made the following comments in an editorial in the *British Journal of Urology*:

> The concept of active surveillance with selective therapy is taking root, and yet there is a paradox. What is respectfully acknowledged at major medical meetings is not, in the daily reality of the clinic, being applied to patients. Indeed, the *proportion of men being managed conservatively is actually declining* (emphasis added).[10]

An example of what Dr. Zeitman is referring to was recently related by one of my patients who consulted a prestigious prostate cancer program back East to avail himself of their advertised multidisciplinary clinic where they claimed, "All treatment options are discussed with specialists from oncology, radiation and urology." On arrival he was shocked to discover that from their perspective, it was already a forgone conclusion that he was starting radiation. The only "clinic discussion" was about how to arrange local housing for the required two-month duration of the treatment. Although active surveillance is slowly becoming more widely accepted, the established custom of treating everyone is still very deeply ingrained.

THE PATIENT'S VIEW

This chapter reminds us how recently prostate cancer treatment emerged from the dark ages. As patients, we are more effective if we know the score. And part of "the score" is precisely how uninformed we are—a lot of men don't even make the connection that a urologist is a surgeon.

When we are diagnosed, the fear sets in; at that moment reassurance is as important as deciding on treatment. It is our hope that men reading this chapter will agree that common sense *is* a diagnostic tool, and that when appropriate, watching and waiting *is* right action.

7.

LIFE IN THE LIBIDO-FREE ZONE

"Doc, can you chop my Viagra into quarters?"
"I can, Sam, but you need a whole one to get an erection."
"Erection? Heck, I'm ninety-one. I just want to avoid
peeing in my slippers."

—ANONYMOUS

There is a story about an unnamed Greek philosopher who lived some 2000 years ago. One morning, when he was in his seventies, so the story goes, he woke up for the first time in living memory *without* an erection, and ran through the streets of Athens crying, "Free! Free at last!"

It's possible that this ancient Greek—call him "Erogenes"—was experiencing loss of libido resulting from the decrease in testosterone that occurs with advancing age. Nowadays, recognizing that testosterone is the high-octane fuel for prostate cancer, we can eliminate it chemically, hopefully on a temporary basis, by means of a treatment known as hormone blockade.

I was in Los Angeles in October of 2002 when I learned that my PSA had again bumped up, this time to 18.3, and my anxiety was spiking right along with it.* At that point, there was no longer any sound argument for continued watchful waiting or, in the newly fashionable military vernacular, active surveillance. I needed to decide on some form of treatment.

As you will discover when you explore the pros and cons of different treatment options, specialists tend to recommend their own specialties. Surgeons want to cut, radiologists want to radiate, and oncologists mostly opt for systemic treatments that include chemotherapy and hormone blockade. Given my aversion to being sliced open, fried by radiation or

---

* Normal PSA is 0–4 ng/ml; slightly elevated is 4–10 ng/ml; moderately elevated is 10–20 ng/ml; highly elevated is 20+ ng/ml.

poisoned by chemotherapy, it was logical for Mark, as a prostate oncologist, to suggest that I consider hormone blockade. And while this form of treatment does not promise a cure, it will buy you time, years, in fact—years during which, I am convinced, as is Mark, the management and treatment of prostate cancer will have leaped forward

The choice of hormone blockade for early-stage cancer was—and still is—controversial. In the past, hormone blockade was used primarily as a last ditch or "salvage" procedure when surgery or radiation failed. Today there continues to be considerable resistance to using it for the less aggressive cancers. The main objection of surgeons and radiation therapists—and many patients— is precisely that it offers no cure, only remission.

Hormone blockade is also known as androgen deprivation therapy and most recently, by Mark, as TIP, the acronym for Testosterone Inactivating Pharmaceuticals. Practically speaking, the treatment amounts to chemical castration with the objective of eliminating the production of testosterone. As such, it represents a considerable advance over orchiectomy, the physical act of removing the testes surgically. In some ways, we are still emerging from the dark ages of prostate cancer treatment. Bizarre but true, you can still find surgeons in Chicago, Dallas, Portland and L.A. who are prepared to cut off your balls to arrest the disease. I mean, *becoming a eunuch at the beginning of the twenty-first century!* Well, it's a surefire way of eliminating testosterone.

Although I had agreed to go ahead with hormone blockade, I still hesitated. Call it "Refusenik's Resistance." The usual procedure, involving the administration of three powerful drugs—Proscar, Casodex, and Lupron—struck me as excessive, particularly for managing what Mark called my nonaggressive tortoise of a cancer. I am wary of what I regard as a general medical policy of overkill. So Mark suggested a conservative approach to the treatment. Because Lupron alone was regarded as sufficient to prevent the manufacture of testosterone by the testes (leaving only a trickle from the adrenal glands), we decided on the single drug protocol with Lupron, known as monotherapy. As Mark pointed out, I could always add the other drugs if the drop in my PSA was unsatisfactory.

Prior to starting Lupron, I took 50 mg of Casodex for a few days to block the potential for a temporary "flare" in testosterone that occurs at the beginning of treatment. Then, on a stormy day in December of 2002, I received my first monthly 30 mg injection of Lupron. In less than four weeks, my PSA had dropped from 18.3 to 10.3 and I knew that the Lupron was working.

In late summer of 2003, with a PSA that had plummeted to 0.125, I took a three-month "holiday" from the drug. Again my Refusenik spirit was testing the boundaries: the "if-less-is-enough-why-do-more?" principle. But in December, when my PSA had crept up to 1.05, I started the shots again.

Toward the end of my fifteen months of treatment with Lupron, I began to wish I had paid more attention to the array of adverse side effects that can occur in the absence of testosterone. At the start, I was so relieved to be spared the possible collateral damage from surgery or radiation that I failed to realize that *every* prostate cancer treatment comes with a stiff price.

THE LIBIDO-FREE ZONE: CHECKING IN

The rule of thumb is: No testosterone, no libido. Libido has been defined (in most cases) as "a passionate attraction to the opposite sex." Without that attraction, the vast majority of men lose all interest in *potency*, a condition described as the ability to achieve and maintain an erection adequate for penetration. So the actual cost of being without a libido is both physical and emotional, and includes, to various degrees, the loss of passion, performance and pleasure. A great many men live in dread of this condition. For them, no libido means that their manhood is deeply damaged.

Once you begin hormone blockade, your testosterone level descends rapidly, sometimes in a matter of days, almost to castrate levels. I could hardly believe it, but after a few weeks my sexual desire was history. Screenwriter Hal Ackerman got it right when he wrote: "Women whose bodies in the past would have stimulated longing and desire, now generate no more response than the sight of uncovered furniture."

And yet despite all the complaints I was hearing from other men about adverse side effects—mood swings, loss of muscle mass, putting on weight, memory gaps—I believed I had made the right decision. I realized that I could live without a libido—I mean, still have a life without a libido—and I remember thinking that if my desire for sexual activity was the price for arresting the cancer, I was willing to pay it. Up front.

A lot of men will disagree. There is a huge constituency who, as a psychiatrist friend put it "vote with their dicks." Not long ago, I interviewed a powerful former CEO of a Fortune 500 company, a gentleman already in his early eighties, who told me without hesitation or shame, "I'd rather be dead than unable to have another erection!" He is not alone. For such men, loss of libido is literally a fate more awful than death, even when it's part of the price of staying alive.

So what can you do to remedy the situation? Even without a libido, you can restore erections through the wonders of modern pharmacology. You can start taking "Vitamin V."

PFIZER'S MULTIBILLION-DOLLAR ERECTION

Anyone who owns a TV set is aware of the monumental sales campaign to make Viagra a household word. Viagra (sildenafil citrate: compound UK-92480) was synthesized in England by a team of pharmaceutical chemists at Pfizer's research facility in Sandwich, Kent. Phase I clinical trials were conducted at the Morriston Hospital in Swansea in the 1990s with the goal of achieving a defense against hypertension and angina. The results were not promising. However, test volunteers reported getting "unsolicited erections." At that point, Pfizer's people, led by Ian Osterloh (the Jonas Salk of erection retrieval), lowered the target of their research efforts so that although compound UK-92480 had a negligible effect on angina, it seemed to induce marketable erections. Eureka! Rise and shine! The birth of Vitamin V!

Testimonies were soon available from high-profile satisfied customers like Senator Bob Dole and the Brazilian soccer star Pele. Revenues in the first three years (1999–2001) were over $1 billion. Pfizer had discovered an erection-shaped gold mine. Viagra proved to be bigger than aspirin, but not nearly as cheap. A far more affordable, yet considerably less potent product, L-Arginine (sometimes called "the herbal Viagra") is an essential amino acid that can relax arteries and in the process enhance sexual performance through increased blood flow to the penis. L-Arginine will only set you back $15.95 for a month's supply versus $20 a pill for Viagra.

Since 1999, a significant number of determined men on hormone blockade have managed to maintain an active sex life despite their reduced libido. According to Sam Otway, fifty-four, a professional athlete, it's been a no-brainer. "Hey, I've been taking Viagra regularly during hormone blockade, and I get it up like a Trojan!" Way to go, Trojan Sam! However, for every Sam Otway there are guys—myself included—who couldn't dredge up enough desire even to *want* sex. So why take Viagra or Cialis or L-Arginine? I'm sure you've seen the TV pseudo-chivalrous commercial pitch: "When the moment is right . . ." The problem is that for many of us on hormone blockade there ain't no right moment.

What also caught my attention was the warning issued to the sexual gladiators among us—a caveat designed, I have discovered, more by lawyers than by chemists: "To avoid serious damage, seek immediate help for an erection lasting more than four hours," the implication being that an erection lasting, say, only three hours and forty minutes is still cool? Add another twenty minutes, then what? Call your doctor? Your lawyer? An animal trainer with a whip? How about *The Guinness Book of Records*?

Although the four-hour fandango known as *priapism* is rare, the condition, if neglected, can become irreversible and you're stuck with a humongous woodie. Reminds me of the story of the mouse with an erection, floating down river on a lily pad and shouting for the drawbridge to open.

According to my urologist rabbi, Larry Raithaus, however, "When you suffer from priapism, believe me, it's no laughing matter. We have to operate and drain the blood clots out of the penis. Otherwise the blockage creates a situation where lack of oxygen can kill off the nerves in the penis. Then you'll never get another erection."

I asked Larry what were the chances of a sexual life *after* priapism.

"No problem," he said. "We can insert an inflatable prosthesis.* That way, you can still have erections. It won't be the same. More like being a dildo with a human attached." He chuckled. "But then some women think that's all we are anyway."

As for me, at least for the time being, I was okay with my libido-free condition. Hey, Erogenes! What's playing at the Forum?

---

* Technically, this is a penile implantation to maintain a functional erection. The device can be either inflatable or a semi-rigid rod prosthesis, consisting of two rod-like cylinders implanted in the *corpora cavernosa* (the main blood-holding chamber located in the penis and responsible for both making and keeping it erect). The prosthesis can have a mechanically jointed "backbone" or a malleable one that allows the phallus to be bent or pointed in either an upward or a downward position.

BOOBS

You hear the term "male menopause" (aka, andropause) flipped around like a Frisbee these days. Many of the long list of possible side effects from testosterone deprivation more closely resemble what a woman experiences in menopause. They include hot flashes and night sweats, weight gain, loss of muscle mass, memory decline and possible osteoporosis. However, my least favorite adverse side effect from Lupron is breast enlargement, official name *gynecomastia*.

This embarrassing and uncomfortable condition (with or without tender nipples which, when you get them, just add injury to insult) can usually be prevented either with low-dose radiation prior to the treatment or by taking the drug Femara. At Mark's suggestion I looked into both options, but I didn't want the radiation and, well, somehow I simply forgot about the Femara. So in the end I did nothing and before I knew it, there they were—my very own set of boobs, a permanent souvenir from my trek through the libido-free zone.

Mind you, I could always opt for liposuction, or breast reduction, a procedure known as *mammoplasty* which, if done unskillfully, may disfigure your chest to some degree but does handle the problem. With a mammoplasty the surgeon goes in behind the nipples and removes the excess fatty tissue. Medicare will even foot the bill. Yet somehow, breast reduction, done more for vanity than for health, and paid for with taxpayers' money (when I was the "boob" who didn't follow instructions!) strikes me as downright immoral. So no telltale scars on my chest. And no need to come up with some bizarre cover story, like one guy I know did: "Oh these scars? Battlefield surgery from when I took a round in Kosovo." Besides, checking my new appendages in the mirror, I have to admit they aren't exactly what you'd call knockers.

HOT FLASHES, WEIGHT GAIN, MUSCLE LOSS, NIGHT SWEATS AND THE MOODY BLUES

In the literature of serious side effects, hot flashes fail to arouse much sympathy and are likely to be regarded as a nuisance, not warranting further attention. Still, they are experienced by up to two-thirds of men treated with hormone blockade, and 10 to 20% of those men are really upset by the experience—which is some kind of poetic justice since the subject of women's hot flashes has its regular place in men's locker room humor. Turns out, it's not so funny when you're the flasher.

My friend Ben Bogarde got hot flashes all the time. "Then there were the night sweats," he complained to me. "I'd wake up drenched. And boy, what about hot flashes during a business meeting? Right in the middle of pitching a new account for a miracle detergent, I went bright red and felt this incredible wave of heat. I guess I did okay though, because afterwards my boss said, 'Never saw you that excited by a pitch, Ben. It really lit you up! Looked like you were having a *glow job*! Ha! Ha! Wish I could get that aroused over a detergent!'"

As for other side effects, I did not manage to avoid either weight gain or loss of muscle mass. And yet, again, I have only myself to blame. Before I began the treatment, Mark had told me that I needed to watch my diet and go faithfully to the gym for regular exercise and weight training in order to minimize these side effects. However, I am basically lazy and undisciplined, and I told myself I would somehow escape fat-and-flabby. My mistake. Still, I was spared the hot flashes and the night sweats. For small mercies, Lord. . . .

INTRODUCING A NEW CATEGORY: "THE POSITIVE SIDE EFFECT"

To put the best face on it, many men undergoing hormone blockade report being more closely in touch with their feelings and crying more easily. For some guys, the most buttoned-up emotionally among us, this could be considered a good thing, particularly from the point of view of our partners. However, a lot of men are taken unawares by such sweeping emotional "liberation" and find it embarrassing. One survivor told me how, when he felt a crying jag coming on, he would take refuge in the shower, where he would stand under the water bawling like a baby. "I just didn't want Gloria to see me like that," he explained, then added, "Actually, when she heard me crying in the shower one day, she got scared and asked what was wrong. Then when I explained, she was really touched." Chalk it up as an unexpected benefit—hormone blockade as a new kind of sensitivity training.

My emotions have never been buried very deep. But once my libido went south, they seemed to erupt without warning and with little provocation. Emotional tremors were triggered by small moments, Little League epiphanies. Coming upon an old couple taking the sun's rays on a park bench, their gnarled fingers lovingly entwined, left me all choked up. Watching a slender Latina girl, still little more than a child herself, straining to hold up her baby brother so he could drink at a fountain, touched me in a deep way. Bravery in dark moments took my breath away. The sorrows of complete strangers brought me to my knees.

My most wrenching emotional experience occurred when I was up in San Francisco for an MRI. The technician had given me earphones to listen to music. Lying on my back and strapped down in the tunnel, I must have dozed off. Waking, I found myself under a waterfall of Mozart, when suddenly, without warning, there appeared, projected onto the inner screen of my retinas, the faces of starving Angolan children. I'd seen those faces with their huge eyes and jutting bones a few nights before on TV, and they broke my heart. The war had ended but nobody was feeding the children. One little boy gazed at me as the translator spoke for him: "I want to get an education so I can find work and feed my family." He was ten years old and starving to death. Lying strapped down in the MRI machine, I began to weep, the tears running down my cheeks, pooling under my chin, and then I was sobbing uncontrollably.

Looking back, I realize the most positive side effect from hormone blockade was a genuine improvement in my intimate life with Jeanne. I was less self-involved, more present, more sensitive to her needs, her feelings. I think of it as listening with the heart. My typical male modus operandi when a woman was troubled was to offer a remedy, a solution. It's what women want, right? Wrong. They want us to *listen*. And as I got further into hormone blockade I found myself relieved of my usual goal-oriented agendas. I was capable of simply listening, without interrupting, until I knew Jeanne had finished saying what she needed to say. In this unfamiliar hormonally uncharged space, not finding myself driven by my libido for the first time since puberty, I discovered a new depth of emotional commitment in my relationship.

In early May of 2004, I got my final 30 mg Lupron shot. After months of monotherapy, my PSA had bottomed out at 0.05, only a breath away from the magic goal line marked "undetectable." That meant the gland was no longer leaking prostate-specific antigen (PSA) and that in all probability, as much as 99% of the cancer was no longer active. Yay team!

Despite my temporary loss of libido and my newly acquired boobs, I found myself feeling relieved and truly grateful that I had taken this route. Jeanne wryly suggested that I might be ready for puberty two.

THE DOCTOR'S VIEW

Ralph illustrates through his own life experience how profoundly men are affected by testosterone, and what a radical step it is to block the hormone. However, as he admits, with some additional preventative steps he could have minimized some of the adverse side effects of TIP. While most of the side effects of TIP are reversible when the treatment is stopped, breast enlargement is not.

When looking at the profound side effects of all the treatments, whether it be surgery, radiation, or TIP, it becomes clear why active surveillance is the most attractive.

8.

TO BIOPSY OR NOT TO BIOPSY: OPENING PANDORA'S BOX

When I look back on all these worries, I remember the story of the old man who said on his deathbed that he had had a lot of trouble in his life, most of which never happened.

—WINSTON CHURCHILL

As previously noted, the prostate cancer world is run by urologists. Urologists are the specialists primary physicians refer their patients to when they need evaluation for prostate-related issues. To most urologists, a high PSA means time for a biopsy—one step closer to definitive information.

In 2003 I got a new patient, Mr. Rogers, a sixty-eight-year-old business administrator with a worrisome family history—his brother had died at age sixty-four from prostate cancer. By the time I first saw him, Mr. Rogers had already been subjected to prostate biopsy on five separate occasions for PSA levels ranging erratically between 8 and 14. Despite his high PSA, there was no evidence of cancer. We performed an ultrasound that showed that the cause of the high PSA was a benignly enlarged 164 cc gland (40 cc is about average in his age group). All those biopsies were done out of the fear of missing cancer. I explained to him that there were other reasons besides cancer for the elevated PSA and because of his enlarged prostate, I started him on Proscar, the standard treatment for benign prostatic hyperplasia, or BPH. His PSA dropped down to 5.2 and remains stable.

One and a half million men are biopsied every year in the United States. At this rate, half of all men in our country will undergo a prostate biopsy sometime in their lifetime. About one in five will be diagnosed with cancer. The majority will have *Low-Risk* disease, the condition that can be safely monitored. Even so, most will receive radical treatment and less than 10% will be placed on active surveillance.

Very few men understand what they are getting into when a biopsy is recommended. Family doctors and urologists schedule biopsies at the first sign of an elevated PSA, rarely educating their patients about what is likely to follow. Once a diagnosis of cancer is made, irrational fears drive most men into immediate radical therapy, even though *Low-Risk* prostate cancer is not life threatening. Having a biopsy can be like opening Pandora's box.

BIOPSY LEADS TO OVERTREATMENT

Our nation is in the grip of a multibillion-dollar industry bent on administering treatment to every kind of prostate cancer whether it's life threatening or not. A well-performed study published in the *New England Journal of Medicine* compared cancer survival in men undergoing annual PSA testing with another group of men in whom PSA testing was not formally recommended. The study, which involved 76,000 men, concluded that PSA testing followed by biopsies led to early radical treatment but it did not save lives.[1] One commentator argued that the advantage of PSA screening was so small that for each man who benefited from immediate radical treatment, *forty-eight* received treatment that was totally unnecessary.[2]

With these looming risks of overtreatment a number of physicians have suggested that we put a stop to PSA testing altogether. They argue that a reduction in PSA testing, especially in older men, would lead to fewer biopsies and to less unnecessary treatment. Though this may be true, withholding PSA testing is impractical. The medical community has come to depend on PSA testing. It's too late to turn back.

Realistically speaking, however, PSA testing per se is not the problem. The problem is doctors and patients overreacting to the information PSA supplies. The solution is not less frequent PSA testing, but rather convincing physicians to use a more restrained approach to recommending biopsy in men with slight PSA increases, particularly when there may be other reasons besides cancer causing the PSA elevation. However, diagnosing every single case of prostate cancer is of highly questionable value. Many men would simply rather not be burdened with the unnecessary knowledge that they have *Low-Risk* prostate cancer.

BIOPSY CAN BE DANGEROUS: REALITY AND RUMOR

There are additional risks associated with biopsy beyond dealing with the uncomfortable realization that you have *Low-Risk* prostate cancer. Studies show that men can literally be frightened to death by a cancer diagnosis. During the first week after diagnosis, the risk of suicide goes up twenty-two-fold.[3] Heart attacks are ten times more likely.[4] To calm men down, they need thorough education and reassurance *prior to being biopsied.* I always explain two things to my patients before biopsy. First, that *Low-Risk* prostate cancer is common, so common, in fact, that the likelihood of the average man harboring some degree of microscopic disease can be estimated by putting a percentage sign after his age. Second, *Low-Risk* prostate cancer is safe enough to be monitored without immediate treatment. Men need this information *in advance, before a biopsy,* to defuse the inevitable fear that will come with a diagnosis carrying the moniker of *cancer.*

Facing the emotional trauma of an unnecessary diagnosis is not my only concern. One or two percent of men undergoing biopsy have bleeding severe enough to require blood transfusion. Men who have a biopsy also face a 1 to 2% risk of infections requiring hospitalization.[5]

Biopsies can cause impotence. In 2008, the journal *Urology* reported on 97 men and their spouses who filled out sexual questionnaires one and six months after biopsy. One month after the biopsy 41% had erectile dysfunction. Six months later, 15% had persistent erectile dysfunction.[6] The results of another study in 211 men was not quite so grim. Erectile dysfunction was reported to occur in 15% one month after biopsy.[7]

Rumors circulate among patients that the trauma and bleeding from biopsy may even spread cancer. However, studies evaluating the outcome in men tested for cancer cells or cancer DNA outside the prostate during radical prostatectomy—a procedure much more traumatic than needle biopsy—do not confirm this. Even when cancer cells are found outside the prostate with specialized genetic techniques using a reverse transcriptase reaction called RT-PCR, studies show that cancer cells circulating in the bloodstream lack the capacity to invade and multiply.[8,9]

MORE AND MORE BIOPSIES

Doctors know that biopsies fail to spot cancer about 20% of the time, especially in men with large prostates. When an initial biopsy is clear of cancer, doctors often recommend a second or even a third biopsy. Naturally, doctors are concerned about missing cancer in their patients. They don't want to be responsible for a delayed diagnosis. They are also concerned about their own vulnerability to a lawsuit. Unfortunately, doctors and patients alike still have the mistaken idea that time is of the essence. This is true for other types of cancer, but it is rarely an issue with prostate cancer.

INSURANCE

There are additional practical consequences to consider before having a biopsy. Health and life insurance companies balk at accepting men with preexisting conditions. If you are insured through your workplace, a diagnosis of cancer can limit your ability to change jobs because of the difficulty of obtaining or renewing health insurance coverage.

Taking time to weigh the pros and cons before consenting to a biopsy means delaying treatment, and if a diagnosis of aggressive cancer is excessively postponed, cure rates may be lower. Fortunately, aggressive cancer (as opposed to *Low-Risk* disease) shows certain signs and characteristics that can be assessed even before a biopsy is performed. The remainder of this chapter is about using such indicators to help determine what is going on in the prostate before doing a biopsy. If these indicators point to the possible presence of underlying aggressive disease, submitting to a biopsy to get further information is appropriate.

PSA AND PROSTATE SIZE

"The prostate is the only organ that enlarges with age," says Stanley Brosman, MD, a well-respected urologist in Los Angeles. "All other organs shrink and atrophy with time." Benign prostatic hyperplasia (enlargement) or BPH is the most common cause for urinary symptoms in older men. More importantly, BPH induces a rise in PSA, leading to concerns about possible cancer. Elevated PSA is the main reason for so many biopsies.[10] PSA is a protein molecule shed into the blood by prostate cancer cells *and by the normal prostate gland cells*. Therefore, the level of PSA measured in the blood is proportionate to the amount of cancer cells *and also to the size of the prostate gland*. Therefore, in any given individual, a high PSA can originate from BPH, prostate cancer or both. More than half the biopsies in the United States are done for evaluation of an elevated PSA coming from BPH. Ironically, in the course of doing so many random needle biopsies, thousands of nonthreatening cancers are diagnosed.

To counteract the "background noise" from BPH-induced PSA elevation—*before deciding to do a biopsy*—the prostate gland should be measured with an ultrasound scan to determine its size and to see how much BPH is present. If the amount of PSA elevation is proportionate to the degree of prostate enlargement—in other words, if the ratio between PSA and prostate size is in the expected range—rather than jumping to an immediate biopsy, additional PSA testing, scans or urine tests may be preferable (see below).

PSA DENSITY

To make understanding this ratio of PSA to prostate size easier, Jonathan Epstein from Johns Hopkins has provided a method for numerical quantification. He calls this ratio *PSA density*.[11] A high PSA density signals that aggressive cancer is more likely. Here is how PSA density works. Prostate size measured by ultrasound is reported in cubic centimeters (cc), 40 cc being typical of a man in his sixties. Once the prostate has been measured, the expected normal PSA for that individual can be calculated by dividing the prostate size by ten. For example, a man with a 30 cc prostate will on average have a PSA of around 3. A normal PSA for a man with an 80 cc prostate is around 8. According to Dr. Epstein's research, when the PSA is 50% above expected, aggressive cancer is more likely. For example, a man with a 30 cc prostate should be worried about the presence of aggressive cancer if his PSA is above 4.5 (an expected PSA of 3 increased by 50%). A man with an 80 cc prostate should be concerned if the PSA is above 12.

PSA CHANGE OVER TIME (VELOCITY)

Another way to distinguish BPH from aggressive cancer is by monitoring the rate of change of PSA from year to year. A PSA rise resulting from BPH occurs slowly, whereas PSA elevation from aggressive cancer tends to occur more quickly. PSA elevation from BPH usually occurs at a rate of less than one-half point a year. (Fortunately, men with *Low-Risk* prostate cancer also have relatively slow changes in PSA over time.) Conversely, aggressive prostate cancer grows more rapidly, resulting in larger annual changes in PSA velocity. Studies indicate that a rise of two points in one year is a strong indication that aggressive prostate cancer might be present.[12]

OTHER CAUSES FOR A PSA INCREASE

There are other non-cancerous reasons for an elevated PSA such as prostate infections, recent sexual activity or laboratory errors. Symptoms of burning pain with urination, urgency or increased urinary frequency need to be brought to the physician's attention because they suggest the possibility of an underlying prostate infection. In such situations, a simple course of antibiotics may be all it takes to lower the PSA into the normal range.[13] (Ralph had a bad scare when his PSA went zooming up from a prostate infection.) PSA also rises after sexual activity, so abstinence is necessary a day or two prior to testing. Lastly, simple laboratory errors are always a possibility. One obvious first step in validating an elevated PSA is simply repeating the test.

DIGITAL RECTAL EXAMINATION

On occasion, aggressive cancers can be detected by digital rectal examination. Eighty-five percent of prostate cancers occur in the peripheral zone of the prostate, the side of the gland that faces the rectum. Certain aggressive types of prostate cancer have been known to make relatively less PSA than might be expected. So, although uncommon, it is possible to diagnose an aggressive cancer by digital palpation when the PSA is still low. An annual DRE examination is another prudent way to screen for aggressive cancer.

PCA-3

PCA-3 is a relatively new test that measures ribonucleic acid (RNA) secreted by the cancer cells into the urine following manual massage of the prostate. Studies show that the amount of PCA-3 in the urine increases in proportion to both the size and aggressiveness of a man's prostate cancer.[14] Unlike PSA, PCA-3 is unaffected by the size of the prostate. Low amounts of PCA-3 in the urine, say less than 40, send a strong signal that significant amounts of aggressive cancer are unlikely. Levels between 40 and 80 are more consistent with *Low-Risk* cancer. Levels of 80 to 100 and above suggest more aggressive cancer. PCA-3, like blood pressure, body temperature and even PSA, varies somewhat from test to test. An average of several

PCA-3 levels done at six-month intervals provide a more accurate reading than just one test.

TWO APPROACHES I DON'T RECOMMEND

Because prostate enlargement is more common as men get older, some experts have proposed varying the PSA threshold level for biopsy depending on age. For example, for men younger than age fifty, a trigger point of 2 is used. Between fifty and sixty: 3. For men between sixty and seventy, they say the PSA should be under 4, and for men over seventy the trigger point is 5. In my opinion, simply interpreting PSA in light of age provides too rough an estimate for drawing reliable conclusions. Just as with any other physical characteristic, men's prostates vary too much in size to simply make a broad guess based on age alone.

Another type of test I don't rely on is Free PSA, which provides imprecise information. The test works as follows: When Free PSA levels are high, an elevated PSA is more likely to be caused by BPH than by cancer. The Free PSA test is reported as a percentage. The normal range for Free PSA varies from lab to lab but generally above 28% means BPH is more likely. When Free PSA is less than 10%, BPH is less likely, suggesting that cancer may be present. Levels between 10 and 28% don't tell you anything. Even though Free PSA testing is cheap and convenient I rarely use it because prostate size can be more accurately measured with ultrasound. Also, prostate infections are known to drop the Free PSA into the cancer range, confusing the situation further.

SOME FINAL THOUGHTS

Rather than scheduling a biopsy at the first sign of an "abnormal" PSA, multiple factors should be considered. The first step is simply repeating the PSA, to see if a random lab error or recent sexual activity caused the elevation. If a prostate infection is suspected, a course of antibiotics may bring the PSA down.

If these simple measures fail to lower the PSA, further testing with PCA-3, color Doppler ultrasound and/or spectrographic endorectal MRI should be considered (see chapter 14). Imaging studies provide an accurate measure of the prostate size so that PSA density can be calculated. If the PCA-3 and

PSA density are favorable, and if imaging fails to reveal any worrisome lesions, active surveillance with frequent PSA and PCA-3 testing, along with periodic imaging, may be preferable to an immediate biopsy. During the monitoring process, some men might want to ask their doctors about taking medications such as Proscar or Avodart, agents that have been shown to prevent prostate cancer. They have also been shown to increase the accuracy of PSA for detecting aggressive disease when used to monitor for prostate cancer[15] (see Appendix).

PSA is a remarkable tool that has transformed the management of prostate cancer over the last twenty years. However, because BPH is so common in aging men, PSA testing alone frequently gives an inconclusive message. Rather than triggering an immediate biopsy, an elevated PSA should set a risk-assessment process in motion. Rushing to a biopsy simply because PSA is elevated frequently leads to a diagnosis of *Low-Risk* prostate cancer, frightening men into unnecessary treatment.

THE PATIENT'S VIEW

As you know by now, I am no fan of biopsies. Despite the party line that trauma and bleeding from a biopsy will not spread cancer, I have a profound mistrust of having needles stuck into my body to remove tissue samples, and an instinctual fear that a biopsy *can* spread the cancer. As far as I'm concerned biopsies are a necessary evil, but under no circumstances should men allow themselves to be rushed into having one before less invasive diagnostic methods have been explored.

In recent years, Thomas Stamey, MD, the father of the PSA test, affirmed the need for a more specific screening test. So while I continue regular PSA monitoring, I eagerly await the news that there is available a less primitive method than a biopsy to determine *for certain* whether or not a cancer is aggressive. In the meantime, I try to keep my immune system as healthy as possible so it will handle any rogue cancer cells that have escaped the prostate gland.

One thing I remember, by the way, about Pandora's box: once all the ills that affect humanity flew out, one thing remained, and that was Hope.

MEDITATION ON "THE BIG T"

I was waiting for my testosterone levels to rise, I got to thinking
the role of that male hormone in our lives. No question, it's the
el. "The Big T" is all about virility, what "makes a man a man." It's
mary source of our power, creativity, imagination, muscle and life
The science is fairly straightforward: testosterone is a steroid hor-
from the androgen group. In mammals, it is secreted primarily in
tes of males and the ovaries of females, although small amounts are
creted by the adrenal glands. It is best known as the principal male
rmone.

e presence or absence of testosterone directly influences mental and
al energy levels, self-esteem and dominance. It is necessary for the
on of sperm. Oddly enough, REM dream sleep increases nocturnal
terone levels. Resistance training can increase its presence. For men,
ig T determines deepening of the voice, height increase, growth of
dam's apple, muscle strength and mass, phallic mass, the abundance
dy hair, libido strength and—the big enchilada—frequency and
ty of erections.

d then there's the Big T and prostate cancer.

THE CONTROVERSY

tate Cancer for Dummies, a far from shabby resource, puts it in simple
ds: "Natural testosterone makes prostate cancer grow faster." Well, yes
no. As I understand it, we don't know with absolute certainty just
testosterone fuels prostate cancer, or the degree to which it fuels one
's cancer as opposed to another's, or the conditions that invite the fuel-
Uncontrolled cell growth can occur independent of hormonal factors
is not well understood. Cancer is an opportunistic process, meaning
ocess that takes advantage of various conditions including diminished
ritional status, obesity, a compromised or impaired immune system
l assorted psychophysical influences. What we do know is that, absent
osterone, the tumor will usually regress and go into a dormant state.
at is less certain is that adding *excess* testosterone will invariably cause
mor to grow faster.

A Sloan-Kettering urologist put it this way: "We're so far behind in
derstanding the role of testosterone in prostate cancer that there are

9.

THE RETURN OF THE PROD

Pointing at his balls, a little boy asks his mothe
brains?" And she answers, "N

— ANONYMOUS

Seven months after my final Lupron shot, muc
that I was gradually emerging from the desert of
According to the stats, normal testosterone levels
800 ng/dl. By January 2005, mine had gone from (
operational yet, but cause for hope.

I was convinced that with rising testosterone l
someday open one eye, bestir itself, come lumberi
sensuous photo of Jeanne combing her long hair tl
and howl with delight.

For the time being, however, I still found the
stimulating as a rubber duck. Then one sunny after
along the Palisades in Santa Monica, I was pleasantl
self admiring a young woman's suntanned legs, the
curve of her thighs. Not long after that, I had my first

I dreamed I was in a hot tub with Jeanne, and whei
voila! There it was, clearly visible through the water–

I called Larry and told him I'd had an erection.

"Great!" he said. "That means the mechanism stil
overcome any psychological blockage."

"Right . . . only it wasn't a *real* hard-on."

"What other kind is there?"

"I just *dreamed* I had a hard-on."

"Oh, well that's different." He sounded disappointed

Still, I took the dream as a good omen. I told myself
of time.

still some basic steps to be taken. So far, we have only very preliminary observations."

Mark is less on-the-fence. When I asked him for his take on the testosterone-as-fuel question, here's what he said: "When men stop treatment with TIP—which is essentially the same as adding testosterone—their testosterone blood levels rise. As a result, PSA rises, which is an indication that the tumor is growing. If you need further evidence, you can see a tumor grow in the prostate via ultrasound or it can even be felt with the finger after testosterone recovery. So there is no doubt that testosterone can make cancer grow. The question is—how fast? Sometimes the growth rate is so slow that it is ridiculous to deny a man testosterone when his quality of life would be so improved and there is no real increased danger. The whole idea of expert oversight is to monitor the situation closely and determine when the conditions are right to use testosterone and when to refrain."

After all these years of living with the disease, I have come to the conclusion that more often than not, it's the insight and involvement of the individual, even more than the choice of treatment, that makes a difference to the outcome and determines why one man thrives and another doesn't.

FOURTH FLOOR: MEN'S ERECTOR SETS: PD-5 INHIBITORS, VEDS, PENILE IMPLANTS, ANDROGEN GELS, SUPPOSITORIES & INJECTIBLES

What do the stats tell us about recovery of libido after hormone blockade? Well, getting accurate reports is tricky. Most men tend to be skittish when it comes to talking honestly about libido and erectile function—or rather the lack of it. Still more to the point, recovery depends on such variables as a man's age, the type and length of hormone treatment, his life circumstances and a variety of psychological factors.

Losing libido is a part of the normal aging process. After seventy or eighty years, the hydraulics of nature's ultimate erector set are subject to ordinary fatigue and malfunction. And yet I know of one eighty-five-year-old whose self-esteem and his view of himself as a man still revolve entirely around his ability to get a hard-on. He and Viagra are wedded at the hip, till death do them part. If he had his way, the Mormon Tabernacle Choir would chant *Viva Viagra!* at his funeral.

There is no set schedule for recovery of sexual function after coming off TIP. Most men will recover libido and potency within a few months, or it may take up to a year. However, even after testosterone recovery, 25% of men over sixty-five describe their libido as "permanently diminished." Yet even with low testosterone and diminished libido, nineteen out of twenty men report that they can get erections with Viagra, although half of *them* complain that they "really had to work at it" to achieve orgasm.

In their useful booklet, *Preventing the Side Effects of Hormone Blockade*, Mark and his partner, Richard Lam, point out that if you don't recover testosterone production, it's not such a serious concern because replacement testosterone can be "conveniently administered through the skin by application of testosterone gel." I know one man, Ed Greeley, who had such a powerful desire to replace his testosterone that he was super generous in applying the Androgen 1% gel (available in 5-gram tubes at $288.99 a tube). When I last spoke to Ed, he told me he had spent a small fortune on his gel, adding, "But it was worth it!"*

Rumor has it that roll-on applicators and nasal sprays are coming soon!

While on hormone blockade, other men have reported success with vacuum erection devices (VEDs). Using a manually or battery-operated VED, also known as a vacuum constriction device, the average man can achieve a "significant erection" within ten to twenty minutes. However, you need to be prepared for a "cosmetic" side effect: the inflow of blood to the penis, combined with the application of a constriction band can, when used over time, cause considerable vein swelling. And there's another caveat. Be sure to use an FDA-approved device to reduce the likelihood of injury by exposing the penis to potentially dangerous pressure, possibly resulting in what my English friend, Harvey, would call "a crushed willie."

Before leaving the Fourth Floor, I feel obliged to mention an entry from the land of the cuckoo clock: a Swiss herbal product called ViSwiss, promoted as "the only pill that lasts 72 hours" and promising "hot, dirty action." The ViSwiss Web site claims that these magic pills will convert you into a "MOVING SEX MACHINE in 20 minutes," able to "fulfill

---

* Much better prices are available. Formulating pharmacists all over the country will formulate a cream or gel in collaboration with the urologist who prescribes it. For example, a biocompatible form of 20% testosterone in a lipo-gel, selling at $50 for a month's supply, was recently provided for one of my friends by the Burns Pharmacy in Lancaster, CA.

your partner's sexual fantasies with a harder, longer and straightened rod!" Mind boggling photos are included to substantiate the manufacturer's claims. One ViSwiss bottle containing thirty capsules ("Starter's Choice") sells for $59.95, and comes with a thirty-day 100% money-back guarantee. As of May 2009, however, ViSwiss was not ranked among the top ten "Natural Male Sexual Enhancement Pills."

Viagra's success has apparently spawned hundreds of these products, with infomercials running 24/7. A product called "Irexis" is currently ranked #1 (sixty pills for $49.99) and boasts a 98.3% customer satisfaction rating. And even "Enzyte," which, as of this writing, only ranks #9 on the hit list, has allegedly racked up sales of over a billion capsules.

Finally, and contrary to Ecclesiastes 1:9, there *is* something new under the sun. I heard about it from my friend Max, who lives in Paris, who heard about it from his friend Thierry, who claims that there's a brand new product, a blend of Viagra and pulverized rhinoceros horn. "But you need a contact," Max told me. "You won't find 'rhinagra' on the Internet."

"Come on, Max! Rhinagra! This is a joke, right?"

"Thierry swears it's true. It's not exactly FDA approved. Thierry made his *achete* (purchase) from a man in tribal robes who operates out of the back of a black Citroën parked in an alley in Montmartre, though never twice in the same location."

"You actually *believe* this?"

"I hope it's true, if only for the ecological benefits."

"What's that supposed to mean?"

"Mixing half rhino horn with Viagra is bound to slow the slaughter of rhinoceri. You're aware that their horn is a famous virility enhancer and—"

"Okay! Okay. Have you tried it?"

"Too rich for my blood."

According to Max, rhinagra goes for $99 per tablet, and keeps you "hot to trot" for up to eight weeks. My idea of a season in hell.

Because Jeanne and I had been apart so much during this time—she trying to sell our bed and breakfast on Maui, me working with Mark in Los Angeles—I found myself in sexual dry dock with zero inclination to rev up my engine. As for trying out any of the available penile sports equipment, forget it! As far as I was concerned, the monastery beckoned.

IT PAYS TO READ THE SMALL PRINT

I recently received an e-mail informing me, among a variety of factoids, that the average size of a man's penis was estimated at "three times the length of his thumb." Upon acquiring this nugget of corporeal wisdom, I remembered what had seemed to me at the time an oddly exaggerated interest in my thumb by a Radcliffe beauty named Lizzie Oxley on our second date while we were drinking beer in Cronin's. When I asked her why the close digital examination, she giggled and mumbled something about a connection to the "power of intuition." Sounded fishy to me. There was no third date.

In the literature that describes the side effects of hormone blockade, I seem to have missed the warning that substantial shrinkage of the penis is common. And although it did not occur to me to measure my pecker prior to becoming a temporary chemical eunuch, it appears that I am now at least one thumb's length short. Some of the deficits are cosmetic, some functional. Checking yourself out in a mirror at the Y, it's humbling to have to look twice to locate your dick. I find myself, for the first time ever, checking other guys for size. Then there's function: when your dick is below thumb size, you have to scuffle to get a hold on it just to pee effectively.

If I had known in advance about the shrinking pecker problem, maybe I could have prevented it with a nightly low dose of a Viagra or Cialis to maintain nocturnal erections. Or maybe "exercising" my organ daily with a VED would have made a difference. Start the day organ jogging. Or I could possibly have helped the situation by what the Scholz and Lam pamphlet refers to as "simple direct sexual stimulation."

"Sounds suspiciously like doc speak for *wanking*," said my Brit friend Harvey.

Erectile dysfunction commercials are ubiquitous on the Internet. Many of them deal with "getting it up," and play on the "ready-when-you-are" appeal. At least as many claim to give the little critter added length. There are over three hundred "male enhancement" products available today, most of them "herbal," all of them promising "bigger, better erections" and, if the claims made on the ExtenZe Web site are to be trusted, enabling you to "grow a solid 9-inch penis." That's as long as my shoe! But there's no free lunch. It seems that along with your solid nine inches, you may also experience "increased heart rates which may lead to palpitations." So you may want to ask your doctor, "Am I healthy enough for a near-death experience?"

The *British Journal of Urology* recently reported on a contraption called Andropenis—a "penile extender device" consisting of a plastic ring, two extender rods, and a silicon band to hold the penis in place. In a study at the University of Turin, twenty-one "highly motivated" patients increased their average flaccid penis length from 2.82 to 3.72 inches in one year. So much for that nine incher! Besides, according to my prostate cancer rabbi, "You can increase your flaccid length all you want. Your erectile length isn't going to change."

It all sounds too medieval for my liking.

JOGGING WITH EROGENES

Eventually I began to realize that in my case the Prodigal just might not return to any useful degree and that I was possibly going to find myself among that 25% of men already over sixty-five whose libido was diminished for good. To my surprise, I felt quite philosophical about it all. How come? Perhaps because the awareness of my new situation came slowly. Perhaps because I was in my seventies and to paraphrase Oliver Wendell Holmes, there is something to be said for the kind of simplicity that is found on the far side of complexity. I'm sure it helped that Jeanne and I are friends as well as lovers, and that her main concern was for my survival, and not whether I could get a hard-on.

Then the irony hit me: Although my PSA had dropped to 0.05, essentially undetectable, and the tumor had shrunk, I still had prostate cancer. And it had been drummed into me that testosterone is the high-octane fuel for any cancer cells with an undiminished urge to travel, to migrate, to colonize. Yet I had actually been *hoping* that my testosterone numbers would bounce back to 300, 400, the higher the better. Was I out of my mind? It was the kind of paradox Jeanne and I used to laugh about, calling ourselves "the O'Henrys," the prototype O. Henry paradox being the one in the story "The Gift of the Magi," where the husband sells his cherished watch to buy combs for his wife's lovely hair, and she cuts and sells her hair to buy a chain for his watch. I was hoping my testosterone would make a dramatic recovery, and yet if it did, there was a real risk that the cancer might take off, spread to the lymph nodes, then to the bones. Good thinking, Blum!

I don't subscribe to the idea that we men are exclusively the products of our hormones, but the degree to which sexual function returns—or fails to return—after any prostate cancer treatment is a matter of serious concern to almost all of us. Myself, I assumed, included. So I was unprepared for how effortlessly I moved from hope to denial to acceptance over my loss of libido and potency. I can honestly say I'm okay with this new situation, at peace with myself. Maybe, in the end, I'll put on my running shoes and go jogging with that wise old Greek, Erogenes. Perhaps even have T-shirts made, printed with the slogan: *Free! Free at Last!*

THE DOCTOR'S VIEW

A physical trainer once told me about a time when she used illicit steroids to augment muscle mass in preparation for a body-building competition. "Steroids" is just another name for testosterone. I asked her about what it was like as a woman to take large doses of testosterone. I'll never forget how passionately she responded. She said, "I felt *invincible!*"

In my extensive experience of dealing with men on TIP, I have found significant variability in how men react to low testosterone and its restoration. Overall, men fall into three general categories. The largest group finds the experience endurable, but looks forward with moderate anticipation to getting testosterone back. The second largest group is made up of men who are very blasé about the experience. Surprisingly, they hardly feel any real negative effects from having low testosterone. Most of the men in this group, for whatever reasons, have already been sexually inactive prior to starting TIP. The third and smallest group is made up of men who express a really strong subjective dislike for the experience. Two men in this group come immediately to mind. Both had mistresses.

10.

TIP: TESTOSTERONE INACTIVATING PHARMACEUTICALS

Wars are not won by fighting battles: Wars are won by choosing battles.

—GEORGE PATTON

Someday soon, a nontoxic treatment for prostate cancer is going to come along. Perhaps the new treatment will be straightforward, similar to the way we treat precancerous skin lesions by freezing them with liquid nitrogen. When that day comes, all the controversies and conflicts about treating prostate cancer will fade away. Everyone will know the best thing to do. Men will simply take the treatment and move on with their lives. The present reality, however, is that the potential side effects of surgery or radiation are intimidating. No one knows who will end up with irreversible impotence or incontinence. With surgery or radiation there is no going back. It's impossible to undo any harm that may have occurred.

A *MEDICINE* TO TREAT PROSTATE CANCER?

What if there were a highly effective treatment with *reversible* side effects, a treatment that not only worked inside the prostate but also had anticancer effects covering the whole body? Believe it or not, there is such a treatment presently available—blockade of the male hormone testosterone, the type of treatment that Ralph describes in chapter 7.

Another of my patients, Max Leiber, a gentle, self-effacing accountant, first consulted me in May of 1997. He was sixty-four, with an elevated PSA of 12 detected during a routine insurance examination. He had intermediate grade disease in the right base of the prostate with areas of low grade disease in the right apex and right mid-gland. Endorectal MRI showed early spread of cancer a few millimeters outside the surface of the prostate. He started a one-year course of treatment with testosterone inactivating pharmaceuticals (TIP) in November 1997 and his PSA dropped to undetectable levels within five months. A biopsy in September 1998 showed no residual cancer. Five years later, in August 2003, a color Doppler ultrasound demonstrated a subtle, ill-defined lesion in the right mid-peripheral zone, and a biopsy showed recurrence of intermediate grade disease. A second cycle of TIP was started in September 2003. One year later, biopsy of the previously abnormal areas was clear and TIP was stopped. Max continued on observation, and as of 2009 had a stable PSA of 1.67.

THE ESSENCE OF MOJO

Testosterone is the hormone that causes masculinization at puberty. Prior to puberty the prostate gland exists as a vestigial nubbin the size of your fingernail. When the teenage surge in testosterone occurs, the gland expands to the size of a walnut and begins producing semen. This remarkable transformation occurs because the cells of the prostate gland are uniquely sensitive to the presence or absence of testosterone. And because prostate cancer cells are derived from the prostate gland, the cancer cells retain the same dependency on testosterone for survival. Cancer cells can grow and proliferate when testosterone is present; they shrivel up and die when testosterone is absent. When testosterone levels in the blood drop, the cancer cells literally commit suicide through a cellular process called *apoptosis*.

Ever since Charles Huggins discovered the beneficial effects of surgical castration for treating prostate cancer, urologists have followed a policy of reserving anti-testosterone therapy until the development of metastatic bone cancer. Since irreversible castration was the only means for lowering testosterone, a hesitation to use such draconian means was understandable. As repugnant as castration is, the anticancer results are undeniable. Doctor Huggins was given the Nobel Prize for his discovery that castration could cause metastatic prostate cancer to go into remission. Today, thankfully, there are medications that achieve similar or better results.

TIP GETS NO RESPECT

When TIP was invented in the 1980s, doctors continued to adhere to the same old policy—they persisted in withholding treatment until the onset of bone metastasis. TIP for earlier-stage disease was scarcely considered. Bearing in mind that the main interest of urologists is surgery, this is hardly surprising. However, there is another reason the idea of TIP for newly diagnosed cancer has been very slow to catch on. The medical community has wrongly assumed that remission in men with early-stage disease will be just as brief as in men with bone metastasis, lasting only three to six years. This lack of understanding about TIP's effectiveness in early-stage disease might have been understandable in the 1990s, before studies using TIP in early-stage disease were published. Now, however, we know that men who start TIP before the onset of bone metastasis respond well for more than ten years before developing resistance to TIP.[1]

LONG-TERM RESULTS WITH TIP

Being medical oncologists rather than surgeons, and being more impressed by the toxicity of surgery than by its effectiveness, my partners and I hypothesized in the early 1990s that medications powerful enough to reverse metastatic disease should be even more effective against less entrenched, early-stage disease. Our initial experience bore out these suppositions. Jim Taylor, a podiatrist, came to our office in 1992 for his newly diagnosed prostate cancer. His PSA was substantially elevated to 34 and his prostate biopsy showed Gleason 6 disease. Even though his scans were clear, his high PSA made us concerned about possible microscopic cancer outside the gland. Using TIP as primary therapy in that era was highly unorthodox. Nevertheless we decided to proceed, encouraged by the knowledge that treatment could be stopped.

After two months Jim's PSA was down to 0.3. A repeat prostate biopsy in June 1993 showed no evidence of any residual cancer! We decided to stop his TIP in February 1994 and by June of 1995 his testosterone blood levels were back to normal. As of 2009, Jim, now seventy-eight, continues to be under surveillance with periodic color Doppler ultrasound and PSA testing. He has never required any additional therapy and his PSA has been stable between 4 and 5.

Over the years we have seen hundreds of men with excellent responses to TIP. Larry McCoy is a professional musician diagnosed in May of 1996 at age seventy-five. His PSA was 14 with a doubling time of fourteen months. Endorectal MRI in August 1996 showed a small prostate with bilateral tumor in the mid-gland and possible early spread of cancer outside the capsule. At the end of a sixteen-month course of TIP, his PSA was undetectable. A year later, an endorectal MRI showed marked improvement. To this day, Mr. McCoy continues on Proscar as his sole form of therapy, with a stable PSA of 3 and a normal testosterone level of 381.

Tom Fox was first diagnosed with prostate cancer in January of 1997 at the age of seventy-eight. His initial PSA was 33. The prostate examination showed extensive palpable disease. He started an eighteen-month course of TIP in February of that year. After he stopped, his testosterone recovered quickly. He has never required any additional therapy other than Proscar. His last prostate ultrasound in September 2007 showed stable lesions in the left base and right mid-gland. In mid-2008, at the age of ninety his PSA was only 0.6.

We recently submitted for publication a scientific article detailing the twelve-year outcome for seventy-three men who embarked on TIP as primary therapy in the mid 1990s. The average age of this group was sixty-seven. The average PSA was 9 with a Gleason score of 7 (intermediate grade). In most of the participants, the cancer was large enough to be felt by digital rectal examination prior to treatment. All the men were treated with TIP and all seventy-three of them recovered their testosterone when TIP was stopped. Twenty-one of these men (29%) never needed any further therapy; a single course of TIP kept their PSA low indefinitely. Twenty-four men (33%) required periodic retreatment with TIP to keep their PSA levels under 5. Twenty-eight men (38%), rather than continuing on intermittent TIP, decided to have local therapy such as surgery, seeds or radiation. Their local therapy was performed, on average, five and a half years after the first cycle of TIP. Of these twenty-eight men who had delayed local therapy, only three developed a cancer relapse and none have developed metastasis.

TIP, A TOTALLY UNIQUE FORM OF CANCER TREATMENT

Prostate cancer is the only type of cancer so exquisitely sensitive to hormone blockade. Although women with breast cancer also benefit from hormonal manipulation, TIP for prostate cancer is approximately *five times more effective* than the best breast cancer therapy. Compared to other medical treatments such as chemotherapy, TIP works much better and is far less toxic. Other than breast cancer, all the other types of cancer, such as colon, lung or stomach cancer, are completely immune to hormonal treatments. Almost all men treated with TIP experience sharp declines in PSA down to undetectable levels.[2] If they have a palpable abnormality on digital rectal examination, the nodule usually disappears within three to four months.

We know that TIP does not completely eradicate every last prostate cancer cell. Microscopic evaluation of surgically removed prostate glands after eight months of TIP shows that total eradication of cancer occurs only in a small minority of cases.[3] However, studies done in our office show that after twelve months of TIP the amount of residual cancer is usually too small to be detected with a careful lesion-directed biopsy using color Doppler ultrasound.

Our belief is that using TIP as a primary therapy is eminently reasonable considering how well men with *Low-Risk* disease fare on active surveillance. If biopsy-positive *Low-Risk* disease can be safely monitored, why not use the same surveillance techniques to monitor men with TIP-induced, biopsy-negative disease? Criticisms of using TIP as primary therapy for *Intermediate-Risk* or *High-Risk* disease seem to be based more on an unwillingness to deviate from "the way things have always been done" than justifiable logic.

SOME BASIC PRACTICALITIES

The medications that make up testosterone inactivating pharmaceuticals fall into three different chemical categories: LHRH agonists, anti-androgens and 5-alpha reductase inhibitors. Medicines in the first category such as Lupron, Zoladex, Eilgard and Vantas are administered as quarterly or annual shots. They work by sending a false hormonal message to the testicles via the pituitary gland, which turns off testosterone production. The anti-androgens, pills such as Casodex, Eulexin and Nilutamide, work at the molecular level by interposing themselves between the testosterone molecule and the androgen receptor. This deactivates the androgen receptor and inhibits cell growth. The 5-alpha-reductase inhibitors, pills such as Proscar or Avodart, block the chemical conversion of testosterone into dihydrotestosterone, a substance five times more potent than testosterone.

Generally, a combination of these medications is used—one from each class—to attain the most potent anticancer results.

As you can tell, I have seen a lot of men benefit from TIP. One of the advantages is how easily the anticancer effects can be monitored with PSA. Within the first few months of starting treatment, the degree of PSA decline reveals how well treatment is progressing. More than 95% of men with newly diagnosed disease see a drop in their PSA to less than 0.05 within eight months of starting therapy.[2] Fortunately, it's a rare cancer that continues to produce PSA above a threshold of 0.05 after six months of TIP therapy. However, when that is the case, additional treatment with radiation is required. These unusual types of prostate cancer are known to be much more dangerous.[4] Even if the disease is not arrested altogether, TIPs usually delay cancer progression for many years.

READING THE FINE PRINT

So what's the catch? Up to this point TIP sounds like a decidedly superior type of treatment. Basically, there are two problems. First is it may be hard to find a qualified doctor who is familiar with up-to-date methods for administering TIP. Second, even though the side effects of TIP are manageable, they are not trivial. Adverse side effects like Ralph's are all too common. Without attention to diet, notable weight gain occurs. Without regular resistance training and weight lifting, significant muscle weakness will ensue. And perhaps most important of all, while on treatment, the majority of men have a total loss of sex drive.

A loss of sex drive is different than impotence. With medications such as Viagra and Cialis most men on TIP can have erections sufficient for intercourse.[5] The problem is apathy, a low libido. Sex can be enjoyed, but it is not sought with the usual male verve. Unfortunately, there is no known way to rejuvenate libido other than stopping TIP.

These issues—weight gain, muscle loss and low libido—are the biggest concerns. However, there is also the potential for additional side effects such as breast enlargement, osteoporosis, hot flashes and anemia. As dire as these side effects sound, they are preventable with proper medical management (chapter 16).

WHAT ABOUT HEART ATTACKS?

Of even greater concern are claims from retrospective studies stating that TIP causes more heart attacks.[6,7] The weakness of these retrospective studies is their failure to account for the well-known fact that urologists generally reserve TIP for men who can't have surgery, those most likely to have pre-existing heart problems. However, there is a single prospective study that also argues for an increased risk of heart attacks with TIP.[8] Offsetting this are higher quality prospective studies that either show no increased risk[9,10,11] or an actual *reduction* in the risk of heart attacks.[12] The question arises as to why researchers would be suspicious that TIP could induce heart attacks in the first place. The reason is the weight gain that so commonly accompanies treatment with TIP. Putting on weight exacerbates diabetes, a condition that is well known to be associated with an increased incidence of heart attacks.[13,14]

How then can we explain studies that report a *reduction* in heart attacks? The mechanism is the very same one that enables women to live five years longer than men. Women have fewer heart attacks because their blood is thinner and flows more freely, creating less trauma to the vasculature. Testosterone in men thickens the blood by increasing the number of red blood cells, putting a greater strain on their hearts and blood vessels. The advantage of having greater numbers of red cells is that physical performance and endurance are enhanced. Nevertheless, at the same time, this thicker blood creates excess wear and tear on the walls of the blood vessels, leading to hardening of the arteries and more heart attacks and strokes at a younger age. *When TIP lowers the testosterone levels, it thins the blood down into the female range.*[15] The controversies raging about TIP's potential cardiac effects are rooted in the undeniable fact that weight gain and secondary diabetes significantly increase the risk for heart problems. However, the best prospective study evaluating this question shows that the net effect of TIP is an overall *reduction* in heart attacks by about 10%. The beneficial effect of thinning the blood is apparently sufficient to offset the known increased risks from gaining weight.

FINAL THOUGHTS

There has been no incentive among surgeons and radiation therapists to support research into the viability of TIP as a treatment option for men with newly diagnosed prostate cancer. After all, it competes directly with surgery, their preferred method of treatment. TIP is rarely presented or even discussed as a treatment alternative. Like all forms of prostate cancer treatment, it has undesirable side effects. However, at least men can "test the water" and determine its effectiveness and tolerability without risking irreversible lifelong impotence or incontinence. If after starting treatment, a man feels that the side effects are excessive, therapy can be stopped and another form of treatment implemented.

THE PATIENT'S VIEW

It amazes me that, even to this day, testosterone inactivating pharmaceuticals are still primarily utilized as a "salvage technique" for advanced cancers—meaning, you have been through surgery or radiation and the cancer has returned. Now, however, thanks in good measure to Mark's unwavering commitment, that is changing. TIP is slowly becoming recognized by physicians—and even more to the point, by patients—as a viable, noninvasive alternative to surgery or radiation. Yes, there are the side effects we could do without, but that's small potatoes compared with the advantages. And almost all of those side effects are reversible. So TIP has been my treatment of choice. It has bought me and my tortoise of a cancer time to wait for less toxic treatments to become available. I ended TIP in May 2004. Since then I have been taking Avodart and monitoring the cancer. But if at any point I need to start treatment again, then I can revisit TIP if Mark and I agree that it's the best option.

11.

INVITATION TO THE "ICE BALL"

Cryo means cold. Cryoablation, cryosurgery and cryotherapy are all
terms for freezing prostate cancer. Cryoablation is done by inserting
probes through the skin between the scrotum and anus (the perineum)
and into the prostate. Cooling substances circulate through the tip of
the probes and freeze the cancer.

— BRADLEY HENNENFENT, MD

Summer of 2005. After living with prostate cancer for sixteen years, my
dread of biopsies had only increased. Both of my previous biopsies had
been bloody and painful, and in spite of repeated assurance that there
was no risk of spreading the cancer by "tampering," I still believed it was a
real possibility. However, my PSA had begun to creep up again, and so at
Mark's recommendation, I was scheduled for a third biopsy, this one with
Dr. Duke Bahn up in Ventura. The procedure was to determine whether
the cancer was still in remission.

I liked Dr. Bahn—the "Duke"—and, more to the point, I trusted him.
Partly it was a gut reaction, but I also knew that he was a pioneer in the
field of cryosurgery, and I was influenced by the fact that Mark referred
patients to him regularly, even though he was a distance away from Los
Angeles. This time, to my relief, the biopsy procedure was no more stressful than a series of pinpricks. And yet, grateful as I was for the Duke's skill,
I still worried all weekend, waiting for the results.

The call came first thing Monday morning. Picking up the phone I
heard the familiar, Korean-accented English, "This is Dr. Bahn. We have
results of your biopsy—"

"Excuse me, Dr. Bahn," I interrupted. "Could you hold for a moment
while I get rid of another call?"

"Okay, sure."

There was no other call. But my heart was pounding. I had to take a moment and just breathe. I hit the button and said, "Hi, Dr. Bahn. I'm back."

"Well, Mr. Blum, results show adenocarcinoma, with cancer confined to lower and mid-sections, left side of gland. We can perform partial cryo. Freeze only the half where the cancer is. That way, preserve quality of life."

There was, he assured me, no urgency. Besides, his schedule was full at the moment. Dana, his office manager, would call later to schedule the procedure. I thanked him and hung up. Then I just sat there, stunned.

Preserve quality of life.

In the 1990s, working with his teacher, Dr. Fred Lee, at the Crittenten Hospital in Rochester, Michigan, the Duke helped to develop cryosurgery. But that was total cryo, freezing the entire prostate, virtually guaranteeing impotence. With focal or partial cryo, the likelihood of impotence is far less, only one in ten. The Duke was one of only a handful of doctors doing partial cryo, which was just beginning to gain acceptance and required extensive experience and training by the surgeon. However, the Duke had performed this new procedure only a couple of dozen times and although he already had a stellar reputation, the idea of being part of his learning curve made me a bit nervous. I was grateful that I had time to think about it. Then, that same afternoon, Dana rang to tell me that another patient had canceled at the last moment, so there was a space available in Dr. Bahn's schedule on Thursday.

"You mean *this* Thursday?"

"Yes, I know, it's sudden," she said apologetically. "But there isn't another opening until the end of October."

WHEN IT'S TIME TO CALL HOME

I told Dana I'd get back to her. I needed to talk with Jeanne before making a decision as potentially life changing as this one, and Jeanne was still on Maui. When I got her on the phone, she listened quietly while I explained, and then said, "It sounds okay. Freeze half of it, protect the rest. You're done with the cancer, and we might still have a sex life." *God willing and the creeks don't rise.* Either way, her calm, reasonable voice was just what I needed to hear. Only then she asked, "And how many times has Dr. Bahn performed the partial?"

"Almost thirty. But he assured me that all the procedures had been successful."

Jeanne said, "I totally trust your instincts, babe. The partial cryo sounds like a reasonable compromise. And you like Dr. Bahn. You'll know what's right for you. I support whatever you decide."

Suddenly I'd had enough of living with cancer. I wanted to go for a cure. With luck, the partial cryo would be far less damaging than any of the other radical, invasive procedures. And Mark approved, pointing out that I'd still have half my prostate in working order. I rang Dana back, swallowed hard and said, "I'll take that opening."

After that, things moved fast. A meeting with the urologist who would be assisting Dr. Bahn—I'll call him Dr. Cleary—was scheduled for the following afternoon. Pre-op was set for Wednesday morning, with surgery at 8:00 AM on Thursday. The procedure would take two hours; I'd be up and walking two hours after that. They'd keep me overnight for observation and, unless there was some unforeseen complication, I'd be on my way home by noon.

Monday night was bad. I awoke before dawn in a cold sweat, still uneasy about my decision. So uneasy, in fact, that I nearly called the Duke's office to cancel. But I didn't.

On the drive to Ventura I wondered why it was necessary for me to see a urologist. After all, Dr. Bahn would be doing the procedure, which involved no cutting. But I told myself that any urologist he teamed up with would be good at his job.

AN AUDIENCE WITH *HOMO UROLOGO*

Dr. Bahn's office was light and airy, with a friendly staff and fresh flowers in the waiting room, but Cleary's office was stark, the walls painted dull gray and hung with a few framed sporting prints. There were no flowers and I was the only patient.

The sliding glass windows separating the office from the waiting room were closed. Behind them, in deep conversation, stood two women, their expressions grim as they stared at me through the glass. One of them opened the window, called "Mr. Blum?" and handed me a clipboard with forms to fill out. After I completed the forms, the other woman, apparently Cleary's nurse, who I will call Bernice, showed me into an examination room and told me to have a seat. My attempt at conversation was met with silence. Bernice walked out, closing the door firmly behind her. I hate it when they close the door.

My appointment was for four o'clock. It was nearly five when Cleary showed up. A tall man in his forties, trim, with dark hair, he shook my hand without making eye contact, glanced briefly at his clipboard and began asking questions. For some reason, he didn't have any of my records.

"As you probably know, problems can arise," he said, looking me in the eye for the first time. "After surgery, there will be pain in the perineum and scrotal area. We'll give you pain pills for that. You may experience bleeding and possible infection of the skin or urinary tract. Swelling and bruising of the penis and scrotum are to be expected because blood oozing from around the prostate drains down the tracks created by the cryo tubes that are inserted into the scrotum and base of the penis."

He handed me a pamphlet titled "Cryoablation of the Prostate," and said, "There's usually sloughing of the prostate material, causing urinary retention, which is why we insert a Foley catheter while you're unconscious. In some cases, we use a suprapubic tube—"

"A *what*?"

"A catheter through the lower abdomen which inserts directly into the bladder. But only if the need arises . . ."

Glancing down the page I was holding, I cringed as I read: "Sometimes the scrotum and penis actually turn dark blue and can enlarge two to three times their normal size."

Cleary continued to describe the procedure: two hours on the table, a spinal anesthesia, freezing probes inserted directly into the prostate through the skin. Argon gas at 200 degrees below zero . . . It was too much. I could barely follow what he was saying.

"Any questions so far?"

Yeah, how do I get out of here! To slow things down, I said, "The argon gas, it says here, that's what creates the ice bubble over the target area?"

"Ice *ball*," he corrected me. "We call it an ice ball."

At one point, when I managed to say that Dr. Bahn hadn't made the procedure seem so fraught with peril, Cleary snapped, "Dr. Bahn always glosses over the difficulties. 'Everything will be fine' is his attitude. My business is to inform you of the potential problems."

Then he really got rolling, warning me that permanent urinary incontinence occurred in 2 to 4% of patients; that a "cystoscopy"—to make sure the urethra is intact—might be required, or "surgical resectioning" (no explanation). And then there was a possibility of "pulmonary embolisms," blood clots that could travel to the lungs.

I stopped listening. My eyes drifted down to the thirteen complications listed in the cryoablation fact sheets. There would be thirteen!

Complication #12 was the final straw: *Failure to cure the prostate cancer.* "It says here that the cancer can come back."

Cleary looked at me sharply and said, "There's a thin strip of original prostate left to protect the urethra, and the cancer can come back there. That's why we monitor—"

"Excuse me," I interrupted, "I need to go to the john."

Clutching the pamphlet, I hurried from the room. What did he mean by "thin strip of the original prostate?" Was that his idea of half? Locked in the lavatory and leaning against the wall, I read Complication 13: *Impotence—Virtually 100%.*

SOMETHING IS SERIOUSLY WRONG HERE

When I returned to the examination room, Cleary greeted me with, "Please drop your trousers." He was already snapping on a rubber glove and greasing his index finger with K-Y Jelly. He took so long doing the digital that I had to steel myself not to flinch. By the time I pulled up my trousers, I was furious. I finally knew what was wrong. As calmly as I could, I said, "Are you aware, doctor, that this is *not* a total cryo? That it's a *partial* I'm here for?"

His blank look told me that he had no idea that he had been preparing me for the wrong procedure! And yet a mistake of that enormity didn't seem to faze him. There was no apology, no attempt to reassure me.

"I prefer to do the total for obvious reasons," was all he said.

I waited for him to explain. What reasons? Better cure rates? Easier to perform? Didn't he understand that my goal was *not* to lose potency? Apparently the 100% impotence rate with total cryo was irrelevant to him.

Suddenly the interview was over.

Cleary was still making notes as I started to leave the examination room. "By the way," he said, without looking up, "if you insist on a partial, you'll have to agree to do a biopsy every six months."

What? Every six months until I die?

I tried to slip quietly through the reception room but Bernice was waiting for me, and handed me a form to sign. I was again confronted with the appalling list of things that might go wrong. This time, presumably for legal purposes, I signed the form without even reading it. She handed me the pre-op instructions, and I was out the door

WHO'S REALLY IN CONTROL?

Sitting in my car, I was still seething about Dr. Cleary. As if his bad manners and his Olympian insensitivity were not insulting enough, what really pissed me off was the dismissive way he spoke about Dr. Bahn. How can you trust a man who badmouths his partner behind his back? *I don't want him anywhere near me while I'm lying on my back, unconscious, with my legs spread and my knees in stirrups.*

It seemed obvious that Cleary regarded Dr. Bahn as little more than a technician. And yet it was Dr. Bahn who would actually perform the cryo procedure. While Cleary did the cystoscopy and placed the warming catheter to protect the urethra, Dr. Bahn did all the heavy lifting—the ultrasound imaging and positioning the cryo probes. With exquisite care, he controlled the freezing process, modulated the temperature on each of the probes to mold the ice ball, shaped it and positioned it just so, precisely the way he wanted it.

Finally I got it! Despite his qualification as a surgeon, when it came to cryoablation, Cleary actually functioned as Dr. Bahn's tech. He set up the wires and tubes that go to the argon and helium machines, then tagged and organized them. But the precise moment-to-moment "weather management" was all in the Duke's small, skillful hands. Duke Bahn was the high wire artist. Cleary was his legal safety net.

The following morning, still uncertain about my decision to go through with the partial cryo, I drove up to Ventura for an eight o'clock appointment to discuss my concerns with Dr. Bahn. Maybe I was overreacting, I told myself. Maybe Cleary was an excellent urologist and that's all that mattered. Maybe I ought to take advantage of the opening. Maybe if I didn't the cancer *would* spread. Mark sent me to Dr. Bahn. It was Dr. Bahn, after all, who had encouraged me to do the partial cryo, so I was willing to give him a chance to convince me to go through with it. He'll be doing the procedure, I reminded myself, not Cleary, and you feel safe with Dr. Bahn.

But when I arrived at his office the following morning, the Duke wasn't there. He'd had an emergency and couldn't see me until his lunch hour, by which time I would already have been through pre-op. That did it. I took that emergency call as a sign, and told Dana to cancel the pre-op *and* the cryo.

REFUSENIK'S RETREAT

On the drive back to Los Angeles my inner critic began working me over with a vengeance. The Voice said: *By this time tomorrow, it would all be over. You may have just talked yourself out of a cure. Nice work.*

Prostate cancer is the tortoise of cancers, remember? I will not be stampeded.

But there was this one opening! If that isn't fate! It's not even 10 AM. You can still turn around and get back in time for pre-op.

It's over! No way am I going back. So belt up!

Why did you really cancel? Was it fear? Who are you?

I turned up the radio full blast, filling the car with the Beatles song "Hey Jude" and began singing, "Take a sad song and make it better . . ."

Still, that last question stayed with me. *Who are you?*

I'm someone who sometimes still gives in to his fear, okay? Fear of missing out. Fear of making the wrong decision. Fear of dying. As I drove down Pacific Coast Highway, Cleary shouldered his way into my thoughts— cold, impersonal, determined, a prime specimen of *Homo Urologo.* Maybe the partial cryo would have gone fine and I'd be cancer free. Then again, maybe I'd end up with rectal damage, or pissing down my leg every time I laughed.

Who am I? Someone who's done his due diligence. Someone who's taken the time and made the effort to interview cancer survivors, surgeons, radiologists, oncology nurses. I've explored all the options, and resisted all pressures to terminate the cancer by radical and irreversible treatment. Well, I'm still alive and kicking, with a low PSA and a small amount of cancer still confined to the gland.

Who am I? A guy writing a book to remind men that time is on their side, pleading with them not to act precipitously when they find themselves in the white-water rapids of panic after getting their diagnosis. I am someone who has consciously chosen to live with his cancer for all these years. Only now, suddenly, *I've* gone belly up, blind-sided by fear! I wanted a cure.

Then, at the last moment, something in me said, *No. No cryo. Not for now.* And I trusted my instincts.

So I still had prostate cancer. Big deal. And I really have to thank yet another urologist for being one of my teachers. If Dr. Cleary had been someone I felt I could trust, I would probably have accepted the Duke's invitation to the ice ball. As it was, my Refusenik sent regrets.

THE DOCTOR'S VIEW

Ralph's emotional meltdown, even after so many years of living with prostate cancer, illustrates the shocking pressures that can overwhelm men with this disease. Most men with recently diagnosed prostate cancer are far less well informed than Ralph, and are panicked by the belief that the cancer can spread at any time. Unfortunately they don't realize that the safest approach is always to take whatever time is necessary to ensure that they really know what they are getting into before irreversible treatment is administered.

You might think Ralph knows how to pick the wrong doctors. Unfortunately, stories like this are plentiful. A patient of mine, a writer who I will call Jeff Kendell, now wishes he had listened to the foreboding feeling in his gut. Jeff knew he was being pressured, but the doctor said that without surgery he would be dead within a year. So he dutifully submitted to the radical prostatectomy. Later he found out that the scans done prior to the surgery showed that his cancer had already spread, making removal of the prostate pointless. To this day we don't know how the doctors missed the critical information that was clearly conveyed in the scan reports. "Who can I trust?" Jeff asked me, "I still have the cancer and now my sex life has been ruined." So what can we learn from Ralph's and Jeff's experiences? Patients need to honor their instincts, even if it means inconveniencing a whole team of doctors.

12.

A NEW LOOK AT RADIATION

Nothing in life is to be feared, it is only to be understood. Now is the
time to understand more, so that we may fear less.

— MARIE CURIE

State-of-the-art radiation can control cancer, often without any severe side
effects. Back in March of 1994 I was consulted by Douglas Reedy, a fifty-
three-year-old professor. His PSA was 2.5, having risen from 1.7 the previous year. He had a biopsy showing low grade prostate cancer—40% of his
biopsy cores contained cancer. We treated him with radioactive seeds in
conjunction with a year of TIP and he has been in remission ever since.
At his last doctor visit in February 2009, his PSA was stable at 0.01 with a
normal testosterone level.

Another client, Marc Roberts, a longshoreman, was diagnosed in January of 1996 with a PSA of 34, placing him in the *High-Risk* category.
His father and brother also had prostate cancer. His bone scan was clear
and an endorectal MRI showed no extracapsular extension. He was also
treated with a one-year course of TIP along with radioactive seeds and
additional low-dose external beam radiation in combination. At his last
annual checkup in July 2009, his PSA was 0.07 with a normal testosterone
level.

CURE MEANS BETTER QUALITY OF LIFE

Compared to other options like active surveillance or TIP, radiation and
surgery have one clear advantage: closure. Closure means eradicating the
cancer once and for all—getting cured! In general, I believe that most
people overemphasize the value of closure due to their distorted fears and
misconceptions about prostate cancer's actual mortality rates. However,
when men emerge unscathed from a successful local treatment, quality of

life is better; they can visit their doctors annually and forget about prostate cancer for the rest of the year.

But practically speaking, how often do men emerge unscathed? For men undergoing surgery, Dr. Peter Scardino from Memorial Sloan-Kettering borrowed the term "trifecta" to describe men achieving three important milestones: cure, maintained potency and preserved urinary control.[1] Unfortunately, even in Doctor Scardino's highly skilled hands, a trifecta occurred in only 62% of his patients, even though they averaged a relatively young age of fifty-eight.

The results good surgeons achieve have not changed much over the last ten to fifteen years, even with robotic surgery. The story with radiation, however, is different and continually evolving. Fifteen years ago cure rates with radiation were lower than with surgery and the side effects were worse. It was at that time urologists coined the term "gold standard" for surgery. But ten years ago, with the development of second generation "conformal" techniques, radiation results improved substantially and became more on par with surgery. Over the last five years, with the advent of third generation techniques such as IMRT (see below), cure rates are at least as good as surgery and the side effects are fewer.

THE REMARKABLE TRANSFORMATION OF RADIATION TECHNOLOGY

The remarkable evolution of radiation is due to improved targeting. Radiotherapy in the past was too unfocused. As a result, the dose had to be kept low because imprecise targeting would frequently burn adjoining organs. Terrible side effects from radiation are a historical fact and widely known to the public. Many of us are acquainted with someone who has personally suffered serious complications from radiation treatment. Throughout the 1990s my own policy was to avoid full-dose beam radiation therapy altogether. I only used low-dose beam radiation as an ancillary boost with radioactive seeds.

Radioactive seed implantation, otherwise known as brachytherapy, started to come into its own in the early 1990s. For the first time doctors could administer extremely high doses of radiation that would remain completely inside the prostate gland without damaging the surrounding organs. Doctors John C. Blasko, Haakon Ragde and Peter D. Grimm in Seattle, Washington, helped pioneer the modern techniques that utilize a special template to achieve accurate spacing of the radioactive seeds throughout the gland. Fifty to a hundred and fifty radioactive seeds (depending on the size of the prostate), each about the size of a rice grain and emitting a one-half-inch spherical halo of radiation, are placed so that the whole prostate receives a uniformly high dose.

In the 1970s various researchers had previously tried to treat prostate cancer with radioactive seeds but without a template (the external grid that creates uniform seed spacing). Poor spacing is what caused low cure rates. Unfortunately, twenty years later, when Dr. Blasko's group came along, the previous bad reputation of radioactive seeds slowed the willingness of doctors to adopt this new technology. Eventually ten-year results confirming that the cure rates were on par with surgery led to more physicians recommending seeds.[2] Finally in 2004, fifteen-year outcomes were reported with good results.[3] Seed implant radiation has proved in principle that properly targeted, high-dose radiation can consistently cure prostate cancer.

HITTING THE BULL'S-EYE EVERY TIME

But let's return to the story of external beam radiation, a craft that has been evolving rapidly over the last decade. Anyone visiting a modern radiation therapy facility quickly understands the absolute importance of targeting radiation properly. To receive treatment you are ushered into a special lead-lined room dominated by a twelve-foot-high piece of equipment that will be targeted on your crotch. It doesn't require a great imagination to realize how much havoc inaccurate treatment can cause!

Better targeting has enabled doctors to reduce the width of the radiation beam to mere millimeters more than the external dimensions of the prostate gland. Radiation exposure to the surrounding structures like the bladder and the rectum is dramatically reduced. This greater accuracy in targeting has also allowed radiation therapists to increase the radiation dose to a range that can consistently control cancer. Moreover, researchers have also developed computerized technology to modulate the intensity of the beam, not surprisingly called intensity modulated radiation therapy or IMRT for short. With IMRT the radiation beam can be "shaped" to match a spherical target like the prostate, limiting "overspray" of radiation into the sensitive surrounding organs like the rectum and bladder.

AVOIDING COLLATERAL DAMAGE

We first became aware of IMRT in 2000 when Memorial Sloan-Kettering reported an unusually low incidence of rectal burns (termed proctitis) compared to older, second-generation conformal radiation technology. The differences were dramatic. One out of seven men treated with older, conformal radiation suffered severe rectal burns. With IMRT, this rate was reduced to less than one out of twenty-five.[4] Back then there were only a few centers in the country using IMRT. We realized that a new era was upon us when the patients we referred to Cleveland or New York returned a few months later gushing about the wonderful vacation they had while getting IMRT. The treatments were administered as a twenty-minute daily visit so most of their time was spent touring around the surrounding countryside, enjoying themselves.

SEEDS, IMRT OR BOTH?

Generally, when an individual is eligible for either seed implantation or IMRT, I lean toward seeds. With seeds, the radiation dose is higher (perhaps giving slightly better cure rates). Also, the radiation does not have to pass through other organs like the bladder or rectum on its path to the prostate, as is the case with IMRT. Seeds are implanted in a one-time visit whereas IMRT requires daily visits to a specialized facility for two months. However, not all men are candidates for seeds. Men with prostate glands over 60 cubic centimeters, and men who have preexisting urinary symptoms as determined by the AUA questionnaire* are more likely to have long-term problems with their urinary tract. Men with even larger prostate glands, say over 80 to 100 cc, or men with unusually severe preexisting urinary symptoms, are also at increased risk for rectal or urinary complications from IMRT.

---

* The widely used AUA questionnaire yields a numerical score. A score above 10 is considered too high to recommend seed implantation.

The determination of whether to use seeds, IMRT or a combination, like all treatment decisions, is influenced by a man's risk category. Men with *High-Risk* disease may be better off with a *combination* of IMRT and seeds because IMRT can be administered to a slightly broader field, creating a bigger margin around the gland. Also, adding seeds to IMRT intensifies the radiation dose *inside* the gland, possibly enhancing cancer control rates.

In men with *Very High-Risk* disease* (i.e., with confirmed cancer outside the prostate in the seminal vesicle), full-dose IMRT without any seed implant is best because there is no established policy for putting permanent radioactive seeds into the seminal vesicle. Full-dose IMRT without seeds is probably also best for men who have documented spread through the capsule of the prostate (termed stage C or T3 in the older staging terminology).

There is another rare form of *Very High-Risk* disease besides seminal vesicle invasion or extracapsular spread: metastasis to lymph nodes (known as stage D1 in the older terminology). Cancer spread to lymph nodes was much more common in the early 1990s before PSA screening became widespread. During those times, radiation was routinely administered to both the prostate and the lymph nodes. Well-designed studies performed in that era proved that extending the radiation field to cover the lymph nodes improved cure rates. Unfortunately, the older technology also increased the risk of damage to the intestines, creating symptoms similar to irritable bowel syndrome. So the policy of radiating lymph nodes fell out of favor. However, thanks to improved targeting, radiation to the nodes with IMRT can now be accomplished with far less likelihood of intestinal damage (see chapter 24).

NOW FOR THE DOWNSIDE

Despite these advantages, even the best modern radiation can cause devastating side effects. The possibilities of impotence, proctitis and long-term urinary problems are real. Side effects of this magnitude are only palatable

---

* *High-Risk* signals an increased likelihood of microscopic metastatic spread outside the prostate gland. *Very High-Risk* disease is the situation where spread is no longer a possibility or a probability; *it is a fact established by scan or biopsy.*

when considered in comparison to surgery. For example, by dodging surgery and doing radiation, you avoid general anesthesia and the risk of blood clots, infections and heart attacks. Moreover, routine prostate surgery carries a one in two hundred chance of death.[5] Like surgery, radiation can cause impotence, but unlike surgery, impotence with radiation is often delayed for several years. Also unlike surgery, radiation rarely causes incontinence.

Each form of radiation has its own drawbacks. Ten percent of men undergoing seed implantation have to deal with urinary symptoms of frequency, urgency, painful urination and slow urination, conditions lasting for up to two years. Infrequently, IMRT causes a serious burn in the rectum. This dreaded complication was far more common in the 1990s with the older technology. Now with the advent of IMRT, the risk is reduced to somewhere between 2 and 4%.

A few brief words about another type of beam radiation called proton therapy. Proton therapy is offered only in a few specialized centers, though new centers are presently under construction. Proton therapy was a very significant improvement over the older radiation technology of the 1990s. However, the most important quality-of-life question when considering any form of beam radiation is, What is the real likelihood of serious proctitis, the type of rectal burn that permanently ruins your quality of life? The only published report I could find suggested a rate of 8%,[6] almost twice as high as with IMRT. However, this statistic is from the mid-1990s. Most radiation experts that I queried believe that the risk of proctitis from proton therapy is about the same as that of IMRT.

BOTTOM LINE: TELL ME WHAT WORKS BEST

Any discussion about radiation being less toxic than surgery is only meaningful if the cure rates with radiation are equal or better. What do the studies say in this regard? When you look at the scientific literature, you quickly discover there are no randomized prospective studies comparing surgery and radiation head to head. Why? Accurate comparisons require volunteers to take one or the other treatment based on a coin flip. As you might expect, it's difficult to find individuals willing to participate in this kind of study.

The cure rates reported in studies are affected by two things: the quality of the treatment and the average *Risk-Type* of the participants. The problem with retrospective studies is that their accuracy is limited by varia-tions in the *Risk-Types* at the different institutions. Doctors studying this matter do their best to match the risk categories from institution to institu-tion, but for a variety of reasons the matching process is less than perfect, since it introduces uncertainty into the conclusions drawn from retrospec-tive trials. Even so, retrospective studies are all we have.

One of the most prestigious surgical centers in the world is at Johns Hopkins University, the place where Patrick Walsh invented the mod-ern form of prostate surgery. Dr. Walsh published his fifteen-year results of surgery in 2007 in the journal *Urology*.[7] The cure rates for *Low-Risk*, *Intermediate-Risk* and *High-Risk* disease were 85, 63 and 40% respectively.

The most prestigious seed implant center in the world is in Seattle, and is headed up by John Blasko and Peter Grimm. These doctors published their results in the *International Journal of Radiation Oncology*, also in 2007.[8] The cure rates were 86, 80 and 68% for *Low-*, *Intermediate-* and *High-Risk* disease respectively.

Dr. Grimm has put together an analysis of the cure rates from twelve institutions using surgery. He also compiled the results from twenty-four institutions using seed implants. The average cure rates are presented in Table 4. Overall the cure rates seem consistently higher with seed im-plants than with surgery.

Table 4: Comparison of Cure Rates Between Institutions

Risk	Surgery	Seed Implants
Low	85%	95%
Intermediate	70%	85%
High	40%	75%

Why would seed implants have superior cure rates compared to sur-gery? One argument propounded by surgeons is that relapses from radi-ation are delayed compared to those from surgery. A study from Johns Hopkins supporting this view concludes that relapses after surgery occur *five years earlier* than relapses from seed implants. This is because a relapse from surgery can be detected at a lower PSA level of say 0.4. On the other hand, a seed implant relapse is generally detected when the PSA rises up to 2 or 3. According to this study, comparing cure rates between surgery and radiation, without a correction factor for the time lag, makes seed implants appear superior.

Another potential explanation for the higher reported cure rates is that seed implants simply work better than surgery. The prostate is located so close to the bladder and rectum that surgeons are able to obtain only a few millimeters of clearance around the gland when they remove it. Inevitably, with such close tolerances, small amounts of cancer can easily be left behind after the operation, a situation called a positive margin, which was discussed in chapter 4. With seed implants, control of the cancer may be more likely because the radiation field extends slightly outside the capsule, thus ensuring against the possibility of extracapsular cancer spread.

THE PROSTATE ONCOLOGIST'S TAKE

After men consult with a surgeon and a radiation therapist and hear conflicting opinions, they are often undecided about what to do. As a medical oncologist without a vested interest in either approach I am frequently asked to act as the tiebreaker. However, even my treatment recommendations are complicated by the multiple factors outlined in this chapter, factors that vary from individual to individual. But attempting to hold all these variables stable, and realizing that the studies comparing surgery with radiation are far from perfect, I can't help but conclude that for most men, one of the two modern radiation options—either permanently implanted radioactive seeds or intensity modulated radiation therapy—is at least as effective as surgery at curing the disease. More importantly, because men live for decades after treatment, it appears clear that both seeds and IMRT are associated with a significantly lower risk of long-term toxicity.

THE PATIENT'S VIEW

Radioactive seed implantation, IMRT and nerve-sparing surgery— each of these relatively new technologies still has its drawbacks, and these drawbacks (well named "collateral damage") can range from wearing diapers, to no more erections, to having cancer left behind. I must say, however, that I know a number of men who have opted both for seeds and for IMRT, and are delighted with the results. Still, it's about tough choices, and living with the consequences. At such times, what a blessing it is to have a knowledgeable partner or a medical expert you trust in your corner. It's unfortunate that medical oncologists who specialize in treating prostate cancer are almost as rare as hen's teeth.

13.

NIKOLA TESLA'S MAGICAL MYSTERY MACHINE

Nature and Nature's laws lay hid in night: God said, "Let Tesla be,"
and all was light.

—AMERICAN INSTITUTE OF ELECTRICAL ENGINEERS
ANNUAL MEETING, 1917

As soon as I stepped off the elevator, even before I'd gotten my first glimpse of the "Giant Tesla," the *thwump thwump thwump* of its coolant system booming down the white corridor hit me like a pile driver's blows. Then I realized: They're going to insert a recording terminal up my butt, strap me down and send me gliding down the tunnel, into the "Tesla-3"—an 8-inch radio telescope connected to a 5-ton magnetic scanner, the first of its kind in the world that performs this state-of-the-art prostate spectrographic MRI procedure.

There is a certain grandeur about the procedure's very name: *Magnetic Resonance Imaging.* The technology leaps over the art of the X-ray, employing radio waves and a strong magnetic field to generate clear and detailed pictures of your internal organs and tissues. And all of it made possible by the amazing inventions of Nikola Tesla who, as it happens, was my boyhood hero.

It was autumn 2005, and I was back in San Francisco at the Center for Molecular and Functional Imaging at China Basin. My goal was clear enough: to confirm whether the cancer had escaped, broken out of the gland.

BRIEFING BY JOHN KURHANEWICZ, PhD,
WRANGLER OF THE GIANT TESLA

It was four years earlier, in June 2001, shortly after my Cipro scare, that I first flew to San Francisco to see radiologist John Kurhanewicz and get a fix on the cancer. At that time, John was still using the Tesla-1.5, the predecessor of the Giant Tesla. Here's what he told me then about what could be learned from the procedure.

"The metabolic information we can harvest is what's crucial. In the areas where there is cancer, the normal product of the gland, citrate, is greatly reduced or not present at all. Another substance, choline, an essential building block for rapidly growing cells, is present in high concentration. So where there's cancer, the choline goes up, the citrate goes down. We graph all the peaks, and we get a real-time snapshot of the cancer's metabolism. The profile of these substances provides a chemical signature for cancerous tissue. That removes some of the ambiguity for interpreting MRI scan results."

A chemical profile from an MRI—that's progress. But it's only half the story.

"What we do next," John told me, "is we go to the old pathology literature: the bigger the tumor, the higher the tumor grade, the more likely it has metastasized. So we take the same concept and apply it to imaging. We say, okay, if there's a major imaging abnormality, and the metabolic changes that we see are extensive and correspond to that abnormality, then we know we have an aggressive tumor. Next we take and combine that information with what we call high specificity criteria for assessing whether the tumor has spread outside the gland. Things like bulging of the capsule, asymmetry of the prostate—there's a whole series of different published criteria. Finally, you add it all together, and you come up with a prediction. It's still only a prediction, but it's a prediction in which you can have a good bit of confidence."

Now, in September 2005, I would be inserted into the Giant Tesla, with its higher resolution and increased magnetic field strength.

I crossed myself and said a prayer of gratitude for Medicare, Tesla and John Kurhanewicz.

CHINA BASIN, HOME OF THE GIANT TESLA

Following instructions, I had prepared myself for the MRI: I fasted for twenty-four hours, drank only water that morning and gave myself the first of two Fleet enemas, because stool in the rectum would interfere with the endorectal probe. Considering the cost of the procedure, the least I could do was provide them with a clean machine.

At 36,000 feet, on the flight from Los Angeles to San Francisco, I managed to administer the second Fleet enema standing upright in the plane's cramped lavatory. (Maybe there's a new *Guinness Book of Records* category here? High-Altitude-Record-for-Stand-Up-Enemas?) Remembering with a shudder my last MRI experience, I took a Vicodin, a mild narcotic that would relax me and reduce the likelihood of my becoming terminally claustrophobic.

John's facility in China Basin was only twelve minutes from the airport. Arriving an hour early, I signed in and, while I sat in the waiting room, read the information handout, "About Your MRI." "You will be asked if you ever had a bullet or shrapnel in your body." Okay with that one. But then came the part that troubled me: "You are advised that some patients feel confined or claustrophobic inside the machine, and that you may require a mild oral sedative, IV moderate sedation or even, on occasion, anesthesia." I hardly expected a day at the beach. But IV sedation? Anesthesia? *No way!* To be on the safe side, I swallowed a second Vicodin.

INTO THE MAGICAL MYSTERY MACHINE

"Ralph Blum?" The receptionist handed me my papers. "Second floor."

My heart rate was already elevated when, changed into a flimsy blue-striped hospital gown, I was ushered forward between two smiling techs. With each step, the amplified banging grew louder. I was led through a door and there it was, Tesla's monster machine. Glossy white, reaching almost to the high ceiling and occupying half the room, it looms over you like a space vehicle in its dock—the Giant Magnet.

The techs helped me up onto the scan slide and without explanation went off to tend to something. I hate it when they disappear just before the next step, which happens to be my least favorite experience—inserting the "electronic sausage" up my butt, and then, God help me, *inflating* the thing! C'mon, guys! Let's get this over with!

They were gone a really long time. Lying there waiting, feeling more anxious by the minute, I tried to calm my nerves by coming up with all the synonyms for *butt* I could think of: *bottom, ass, buttocks, tail, rump, posterior, hindquarters, rear end, behind, backside, duff, rectum, fanny, keister* (rhymes with *Easter*), *popo, can, caboose, tush, botto, prat* (as in "pratfall"), *arse, buns, heinie* (That's what my uncle Jacques called the

Germans during World War II, "Heinies"). And since the techs still hadn't returned, I scratched up a few in translation: *derriere, culo, pogue, ketsu* or *oshiri* in Japanese; Japanese women say *oido*, meaning "the part we use for sitting," *zadnitsa* (standard) and *zhopa* (vulgar) in Russian. And the Yiddish, *tuchas*. I've noticed that "anus" is popular with older docs. I prefer *butt*, with the British *bum* as a backup (so to speak), and the slapstick comedy *keister* kept in reserve for those prostate moments when I'm tempted to tell some overbearing urologist where he had his head —.

"If you're ready, Mr. Blum?"

They were turning me onto my side when I felt my mood shift. It was amazing: from one moment to the next I was tension free, totally relaxed, on cruise control. I was only half aware of them inserting the probe, blowing it up, feeling the pressure as it expanded and docked against my rectal wall. Thanks to the two Vicodin, they could have hung me upside-down on a hook and I wouldn't have complained.

Smiling, and with my eyes closed, I was actually feeling a sense of joy at being there, and thinking: *What a hoot! Tesla's patent for the rotating magnetic field made possible this monster machine into which my body will momentarily be sliding.*

"Now over on your back . . . that's it."

Arms clasping me, hands strapping me down, tightening the straps . . . They gave me earplugs and headphones out of which a voice said, "Here we go."

Feeling motion, I opened my eyes. I was sliding into the yawning white mouth of Tesla's giant magnet, gliding along the cylindrical channel with its low curved dome and runway of little lights just a foot above my head, and with only inches to spare on either side of me. Cozy in a way. But God help you if you were seriously obese.

So there I was, trussed up like a pork roast. I had hoped they would ask, "Are you claustrophobic?" so I could answer, "Only when I'm tied up and inserted into a narrow tunnel with an inflated sausage up my butt." Nobody asked.

With no warning, a torrent of music flowed into my ears, flooding my brain with Wagner's Prelude to Act II of *Lohengrin*. Perfect! Let there be no doubt about the Teutonic grandeur of this procedure . . . Then, underneath the horns and the woodwinds, from the Machinery Section, came an *allegro* passage for PILE DRIVERS (*thumpa-thumpa-thumpa-thump!*), followed by a cadenza for MONSTER CLICKERS . . . I was moving again, inching forward. Stopping. Moving. Stopping. PILE DRIVERS . . . CLICKERS . . . PILE DRIVERS . . . then silence.

The high tide of Wagner was followed by eight bars of absolute silence. Then, out of the stillness came the honeyed whispering of Vivaldi, his flute concerto, added to which was a solo for METAL MOUSE nibbling on metal cheese *(tinka-tinka-tink-tink-a-tink-a-tink!)* . . . My body was being sliced into slender images. I was beginning to drift away.

The tech's voice came through the headphones. "How you doing, Mr. Blum?"

"Happy as a pig in swill!"

Well, almost: I had no place to move my arms. My elbows, locked against the tunnel walls, were beginning to ache. I managed to stretch my hands an inch or so along my thighs, easing the pressure. "Once you're inside you'll be able to move your arms," they told me. Fat chance! And yet, thanks to the Vicodin, I couldn't care less. Something very pleasant was happening: a softening and a total sense of ease and well-being.

From that point on, it was all like a dream.

Suddenly, Nikola Tesla is there, standing right in front of me, his rugged face with its Serbian bandit's mustache and dark, brooding eyes projected on my inner screen. Tesla is in his laboratory giving an exhibition to allay fears about his latest invention, the alternating current. Young and passionate, he stands with his feet wide apart, his face ecstatic as he lights lamps without wires by gripping the terminals, one in each hand, as the crackling electricity courses through his body.

THE MAN WHO LIT UP BUFFALO, NEW YORK

Reel back sixty years. I am thirteen years old; it is April 12, 1945, a Thursday. I am just coming out of the big Hawthorne School doors into the afternoon sunlight on Rexford Drive. My English teacher, Miss Lucille Murphy, is calling my name, hurrying after me, red faced, tears running down her cheeks, sobbing, "FDR is dead!" She shoves my extra credit essay into my hands and flees. There's an A+ in a red loop on the cover page over the title, "Nikola Tesla: Magician of Light."

I first learned about Tesla from Miss Murphy, who regarded him as a "flashing star in the scientific firmament." In Beverly Hills, where I grew up, stars were the currency of metaphors. They were also my father's clients. Famous names were regular guests at our dinner table—Tyrone Power, Irene Dunne, Charles Boyer and Johnny (Tarzan) Weissmuller, even Roy Rogers. And although I dutifully collected their signatures in my autograph book, Nikola Tesla, "the dreamer from Similjan," was my only true hero.

I knew his story by heart: How he arrived in the United States in 1884 with less than a dollar in his pocket, a few poems and specifications for a flying machine. How he went on to invent systems that anticipated worldwide wireless communications, fax machines, radar and radio-guided missiles. He had over seven hundred patents to his name when he died, including patents for the fluorescent light, the polyphase alternating current, the induction motor. Edison ripped him off royally. He made George Westinghouse rich. He drank beer and ate pretzels with Mark Twain, who he always addressed as "Mr. Clemens." He worked with time travel technology, until he and Einstein concluded that it wouldn't be good for humans.

And yet despite his genius, he couldn't balance a checkbook or look after himself. Tesla died a lonely man, in poverty. After his death, the U.S. government Custodian of Alien Property impounded his trunks, which held all his papers, his diplomas and other honors, his letters, his laboratory notes and the results of his experiments. His creative output was so bountiful that, to this day, scientists still comb his papers for unrealized ideas. And yet, because of his eccentric personality and bizarre claims, Tesla was considered "wonky" and was denied the Nobel Prize.

What really blew me away as a kid with a nose for justice was learning that two of Tesla's U.S. patents (#645,576 and #649,621) formed the basis for the U.S. Supreme Court's 1943 decision to overturn Marconi's patent for the invention of radio and award it to Tesla. Sadly, when the Court finally ruled in his favor, Nikola Tesla had been dead for five months and eleven days.

So here's to you, Nikola Tesla. Back in 1896, you harnessed the power of Niagara Falls and lit up Buffalo, New York. Now here you are, lighting up my prostate and hopefully bringing me some peace of mind. Well, whatever the outcome, you have my undying gratitude. *May the earth lie lightly upon you!*

FINDINGS

More than half an hour had passed and I was moving again, sliding out of the tunnel, coming in for a landing. For the finale, the Symphony Orchestra and Construction Workers Ensemble offered Holst's "Mars the Bringer of War" from "The Planets" (*Thud! Thud! Thud! Thud!*). Then by slow ticks, I was withdrawing, departing from the Giant Tesla, my prostate observed, its metabolic functions identified, the evidence recorded.

The music ended. In absolute silence, I came sliding back into the light of day.

A week later, the results were in my mailbox. Under "Findings" was the following stark sentence: "No evidence of extracapsular extension." Whew! Thank you, God! I called John, and told him how relieved I was, since what had concerned me most was the possibility the cancer had spread to the seminal vesicles

"Then we've got a problem," he said

"What problem? What do you mean, *problem?*"

"The metabolic data we record only comes from the prostate itself. We can't include the seminal vesicles without introducing contamination and making our interpretation of the data very difficult."

Aw shit! That was *not* what I wanted to hear.

I said, "Then what's the likelihood that the seminal vesicles are involved?"

John told me I was fortunate because my tumor was midgland rather than at the base—abutting the seminal vesicles—so that chances of seminal vesicle involvement were minimal.

Minimal. Not the reassurance I had hoped for.

Dark thoughts came unbidden in the night, and I would lie in bed wondering: *Is there cancer in the seminal vesicles that's just too tiny to see?* Since the seminal vesicles are the staging area, first for the lymph glands, then for the bones, I needed to know for sure.

The Giant Tesla had left me twisting in the wind.

THE DOCTOR'S VIEW

Accurate information about any cancer is essential for decision making. How big is the tumor? Does the cancer penetrate the capsule wall? Is the cancer metabolically aggressive? And even more significant, "Is it growing?" A question that can be answered by evaluating sequential scans. Prostate imaging with MRI is cumbersome and expensive. However, we always judged it to be a good value if a biopsy could be avoided. The importance of imaging, with MRI or color Doppler ultrasound, is further elaborated in the next chapter.

14.

QUALITY IMAGING: A DOORWAY TO LESS TOXIC TREATMENT

In the long run, men only hit what they aim at.

— HENRY DAVID THOREAU

Accurate monitoring is essential for active surveillance. At present, most centers rely on periodic random needle biopsies as their primary form of monitoring. My medical practice was confronted with this challenge in the early 1990s when after TIP, men needed the same monitoring as active surveillance. Back then our preferred alternative to repeated biopsies was the same imaging approach Ralph chose, spectrographic endorectal MRI at the University of California at San Francisco.[1]

TAKING A LOOK INSIDE THE PROSTATE

Most people have heard of MRI, which is used to image various parts of the body such as the bones, the brain or the abdomen. For prostate scanning, MRI image quality is improved by using a probe inserted into the rectum, appropriately called an endorectal coil. Even though the exam can be uncomfortable, it is less stressful than a biopsy.

Spectroscopy is a new enhancement of MRI developed to reduce uncertainty about whether lesions detected on standard MRI are cancerous or benign. A spectrographic MRI (S-MRI) consists of two components: the MRI and the spectroscopy. As Ralph described in the previous chapter, spectroscopy is like a chemical assay that identifies specific molecules that occur in cancerous tissue. If abnormal amounts of these molecules — citrate or choline — are seen in the same area of the prostate where the MRI shows lesions, those lesions are more likely to be cancerous.[2]

Hundreds of our patients have traveled from Los Angeles to San Francisco for S-MRI scanning rather than undergo repeated random biopsies.

Over the years this technology has become more widely accepted.[3,4,5] These days, centers of excellence like Memorial Sloan-Kettering and University of California, San Francisco, integrate S-MRI into their regular clinical diagnostic practice.[6]

IMAGING BECOMES MORE ACCESSIBLE

Our reliance on MRI for prostate imaging shifted when a well-known prostate radiologist and cryosurgeon,* Dr. Duke Bahn (already introduced to you in Ralph's chapter about the Ice Ball) moved his practice from Michigan to the West Coast in 2002. Even prior to his move, Dr. Bahn and his mentor, Dr. Fred Lee, were well known for their revolutionary work developing color Doppler ultrasound imaging. [7] After Dr. Bahn settled in, I made a point of visiting him to observe his work firsthand. I was immediately impressed by the images attained with color Doppler. They easily rivaled the quality seen with MRI. I was also impressed by how conveniently the study could be performed in the office. Starting in 2004, Dr. Bahn was kind enough to teach my partner, Dr. Richard Lam, and me how to use this technology.

COLOR DOPPLER IS STILL CONTROVERSIAL

After seeing the utility of color Doppler, many of our patients question why it is not more widely used. Unfortunately, in the early years, ultrasound imaging got a reputation for poor image quality, and studies conducted in the past concluded that it was inaccurate, missing many tumors that were detected by random biopsy. Regrettably, based on those early studies, much of the medical community still believes that ultrasound is unreliable and of little value except as a rudimentary aid for performing a random needle biopsy. Even though modern ultrasound equipment is vastly improved, there has been little interest in revisiting this technology.

Most urologists who rely on biopsies to monitor their patients are correct when they point out that even state-of-the-art ultrasound can miss small cancers. All monitoring tools—PSA velocity, PSA density, PCA-3,

---

* A radiologist is not the same as a radiation therapist. Radiologists specialize in doing scans and reading them. Radiation therapists specialize in administering radiation.

digital rectal exam, ultrasound, spectrographic MRI or even biopsy itself—have limitations. Color Doppler is only one of many tools that provide useful information about the status of the cancer in the prostate. The goal is not to eliminate biopsies altogether but rather to *reduce their use as much as possible.*

The general medical community is unfamiliar with today's state-of-the-art prostate imaging. Color Doppler ultrasound is really two scans in one: a "gray-scale" image that provides images in black and white, and a color image that detects areas of increased blood flow. Urologists use gray-scale ultrasound machines in their offices to locate the prostate when performing random biopsies. Even this simple equipment is unlikely to detect anything but large, obvious lesions. Color Doppler ultrasound provides higher resolution gray-scale images and also "sees" areas of increased blood flow. Aggressive prostate cancers have an increased blood supply that can be imaged with color Doppler.[8]

BIOPSY STUDIES CONFIRM THE ACCURACY OF COLOR DOPPLER

The accuracy of this technology has been tested in studies by comparing color Doppler lesion-directed biopsy to standard random biopsy. Such studies are fairly easy to perform. Two urologists are needed. The first urologist performs a lesion-directed biopsy targeting suspicious areas detected by color Doppler. The second urologist follows immediately afterward using standard ultrasound to perform a biopsy in a random grid pattern. It has been shown that color Doppler technology, especially with contrast, finds more high-grade cancers than a random biopsy, even though the random biopsy utilizes twice as many needle cores.[9,10]

In my experience, color Doppler images are comparable in quality to S-MRI. But color Doppler is certainly easier to perform than S-MRI: it takes less time, the probe is much smaller and, because it is an office procedure, travel to a specialized facility is unnecessary. The biggest advantage over S-MRI, however, is the ability to perform a lesion-directed biopsy.[11] The accuracy of the biopsy is easily documented because color Doppler can literally photograph the trail of the biopsy needle as it darts through the targeted lesion. The material from the lesion can then be examined under a microscope to determine if it is malignant or benign.

With this more accurate information, patient management, whether for monitoring or for staging prior to treatment, becomes much easier.

AN IMPORTANT STEP *PRIOR TO* DIAGNOSTIC BIOPSY

With access to better imaging, the question arises, "How about using color Doppler to monitor men who have never been diagnosed with prostate cancer?" Instead of automatically consigning every man with a slightly elevated PSA to immediate random biopsy, the information obtained with color Doppler can be used along with other indicators such as PSA velocity, PSA density, PCA-3 and DRE to determine whether a biopsy is really required.

INSURANCE AGAINST LOW-PSA PRODUCING CANCERS

In men on active surveillance the cancers are small and produce relatively little PSA. *Gland*-generated PSA causes major "background noise" making it difficult to interpret PSA changes because the PSA is mostly coming from the prostate gland, not the cancer. With color Doppler, you can avoid this problem by measuring the size of the tumor directly and monitoring its growth over time. On many occasions I have seen enlarging lesions detected by color Doppler even when PSA levels remain stable. Image 1 (on page 132) is a vivid illustration.

This image comes from an elderly man on active surveillance. It shows a cross-section through the middle of the prostate (the two images are the same). The large, black semicircle at the bottom is the rectum. The prostate gland is directly above. The cancer in the prostate is marked by small crosses on the right-hand image. The small spots in the cancer in the *left* picture were red in the original image (black-and-white image reproduction in this book does not show the original color). These "red" spots are indicative of increased blood flow classically associated with higher grade cancer. The significant thing is that another ultrasound from six months earlier (Image 2) *was completely clear of cancer*. In other words, the cancer, which is seen on the left side of the prostate, grew to this size over a very short period of time! *During that same period his PSA hardly changed.* Rapidly growing prostate cancer like this is uncommon. But when it occurs, early detection is essential.

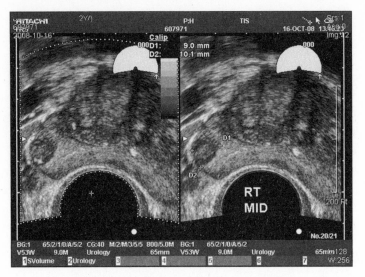

Image 1. Color Doppler scan, October 2008.

DIRECTING TREATMENT AT THE TUMOR

Quality prostate imaging opens the door to another potential benefit: targeted therapies. Why ablate or remove the whole prostate, as is standard with surgery and radiation, if only a small portion of the gland contains cancer? Why not perform a lumpectomy like we can do for breast cancer? In chapter 11, Ralph describes how he came close to adopting this approach for himself. Peter Knox, a seventy-four-year-old retired engineer, is someone who did. Dr. Knox was diagnosed in January 2004. His PSA was 3.0, up from 1.6 the previous year. Random biopsy showed two of twelve cores positive for Gleason 5 + 4 = 9 making him *High-Risk*. Dr. Knox was treated initially with TIP and after one year his PSA dropped to undetectable levels. However, color Doppler–directed biopsy showed persistent disease. He elected to have a focal treatment, cryotherapy that was limited to one side of the gland. Dr. Bahn performed the cryotherapy using color Doppler to navigate the cryo probes into the area of the cancer. The treatment was successful and, at Dr. Knox's last visit to my office in February of 2009, his PSA was stable at 0.985. His sexual potency was intact and his testosterone was normal.

Focal treatment is still controversial, with experts arguing passionately both for and against this new approach. Some claim focal therapy won't work because in many cases men will have other small cancers in a different area of the prostate. The naysayers believe that the danger of leaving

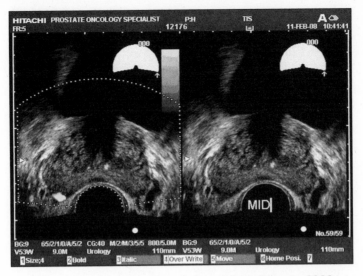

Image 2. Color Doppler scan of same patient, February 2008.

these small cancers behind is unacceptable. Experts who support focal therapy argue that quality imaging and staging biopsies almost always detect secondary tumors that are large enough to be consequential. They maintain that small, low-grade microscopic prostate cancers missed with state-of-the-art staging are unimportant. Furthermore, they ask, why can't selective ablation of the most prominent cancer be performed while continuing with close surveillance of the rest of the gland? If another cancer shows up, further treatment can be administered at that time.

As we learned through Ralph's introduction, cryotherapy is accomplished by circulating argon gas through small hollow needles inserted into the prostate to create an expanding ice ball at the tip of the needle. The size of the ice ball is controlled by adjusting the flow rate of the argon. Originally, cryotherapy was used for freezing the entire prostate. However, the popularity of whole-prostate cryotherapy is limited because impotence occurs 90% of the time. Preliminary studies with focal cryotherapy indicate good cancer control rates and lower impotence rates of around 20%.[12,13]

FINE TUNING TREATMENT TO LIMIT SIDE EFFECTS

There are other practical uses for color Doppler ultrasound. The ability to track cancer progression and regression opens the door to using milder treatment. Historically, aggressive treatment has been deemed necessary to offset uncertainty about the cancer status. A "safety factor" of maximally intensive treatment was deemed necessary to insure against the possibility of cancer progression. For example, before we had color Doppler our testosterone blockade policy invariably consisted of combination therapy with three drugs, Casodex, Proscar and Lupron. As therapists we took comfort knowing that even if we got suboptimal results, we were doing everything possible to hinder cancer growth and shrink the tumor. Now, with the ability to track the cancer more accurately via color Doppler, we are bolder about using less aggressive forms of therapy, such as Casodex by itself.[14] Using less toxic drugs, especially in men who are elderly or frail, is essential for maintaining quality of life. It can also be an important issue in younger men if maintaining sexual function is considered imperative. Let me illustrate this concept with a few examples.

Mr. Treacher, a retired military man, was diagnosed at age forty-nine. He had a random biopsy in July of 2001 showing three cores positive for Gleason $3 + 4 = 7$ disease. After trying a variety of herbal therapies he consulted us in December 2003 and started TIP. His PSA dropped to undetectable. However, color Doppler–directed biopsy in September 2005 showed persistent disease on the right side of the gland and seminal vesicle. He restarted TIP but took himself off therapy after three months because he was falling in love with a woman thirty years his junior. From that point on he was adamantly against any treatment that could curtail his sexual activity. Off treatment, his PSA started rising. Consequently he restarted Casodex and Avodart (without Lupron) with reasonably good results. In January 2009 his PSA was only 0.290 with a testosterone level of 838. His cancer appeared stable with color Doppler.

Mr. Allen, a music critic, was diagnosed with prostate cancer in May of 2003 at the age of eighty. His urologist administered a single three-month Lupron shot which resulted in severe fatigue and muscle atrophy leading to confinement in a wheelchair. He consulted us in October 2003. His testosterone was still low at 63 so we began administering testosterone to improve his strength. He was soon able to resume walking. However, his PSA also rose. We tried a variety of medications such as Flutamide and Nilutamide but they all caused severe fatigue. Radiation was not an option because of his history of irritable bowel syndrome. Ultimately, in January 2006, when his PSA had risen to 13.6, he was started on one Casodex pill every five days, which was well tolerated. As of early 2009 he continues on testosterone supplementation and minimal Casodex with a stable PSA of 8. Periodic examinations with color Doppler show that the cancer remains stable.

These patients' cases illustrate how treatment can be customized according to the specific needs of each individual. Too often, treatment selection is based on the false assumption that all types of prostate cancer are equally dangerous. This assumption goes unchallenged when there is a lack of accurate feedback about how the cancer is behaving. Poor assumptions lead to mistakes. Neither overtreatment, which produces undesirable side effects, nor undertreatment, which allows the disease to progress, is acceptable. When using less than maximal therapy, we must have accurate information about how the cancer is behaving. Rather than relying on periodic biopsies, we have found color Doppler to be an excellent way to track cancer activity.

THE PATIENT'S VIEW

Mark's survey of imaging in this chapter provides a comprehensive, readily accessible overview of the current field, the options, the possible pitfalls. It was from the color Doppler imaging Dr. Bahn performed in 2008 that I learned the reassuring news of the lack of blood flow and stalled growth to my tumor. For men with prostate cancer it is encouraging to know that with color Doppler it is possible to perform a lesion-directed biopsy instead of just randomly jabbing the prostate. And given my mistrust of biopsies, I was particularly pleased when I learned that color Doppler can also provide information that reduces the need for repeated biopsies. What does puzzle me is how rarely color Doppler is used by urologists. As of 2010 there are only a handful of places in California where a color Doppler–assisted ultrasound is available.

15.

NOW PLAYING FOR A LIMITED TIME ONLY: THE COMBIDEX FOLLIES

"Confined to the gland" is doc-speak. And the so-called prostate wall
is no more than a fibrous layer, about the thickness of the rind of
a lemon. You can clearly dissect the capsule off the gland, but the
capsule itself is just a lot of glandular cells compressed. When the
cancer is ready to go, it goes, wall or no wall. And once it extends up
into the seminal vesicles, it can easily be transported to the regional
lymph nodes. *Then* you can start to worry.

— LARRY RAITHAUS, MD, *urologist*

A year after that experience in the Giant Tesla, there was a change in my
status. Duke Bahn's ultrasound confirmed that the tumor had increased in
size, and that the cancer was definitely out of the prostate and had invaded
the left seminal vesicle. My Gleason Score had gone from 6 to 7, the point
beyond which even a Refusenik will begin to have long second thoughts
about undergoing some form of radical intervention.

For the first time since I'd known him, Mark was making quiet references to treatment choices. Hard to ignore when your oncologist/writing
partner is hinting that treatment might be timely. Still, before I made any
decisions I needed to know one thing: Had the cancer metastasized? Had
it spread to the lymph nodes?

Only there was a problem. No sufficiently reliable diagnostic test for lymphatic involvement was available in the U.S. The primary FDA-approved diagnostic tool, Prostascint, which relies on an injection of indium (a radioactive
dye that is taken up by the lymph nodes), can produce a high percentage of false
positives. Not good enough. So once again, I stuck with active surveillance.

Then, just before Christmas 2006, Mark told me about Combidex, the
brand name for ferumoxtran-10, a nanoparticle* of super paramagnetic

---

* Nanoparticle: a unit of matter, a minute particle that is 10^{-9} meter, or one billionth of
a meter. To give you an idea of the scale, a single nanoparticle is 1/50th the diameter of
a human hair.

iron oxide developed for intravenous administration as a contrast agent for use with magnetic resonance imaging. According to the makers, Advanced Magnetics, Inc., Combidex can "assist in the differentiation between meta-static and non-metastatic lymph nodes in patients with confirmed primary cancer who are at risk for lymph node metastases." How it works is that metastatic lymph nodes show less "uptake" of the iron oxide nanoparticles so they remain white, while the healthy nodes are black. In this shoot-out, the "good guys" wear the black hats.

However, although Combidex is significantly more trustworthy than any other diagnostic agent, it has been denied approval by the FDA and is unavailable in the U.S. In fact, there is only one place in the world where, as I write, the Combidex MRI is offered: at St. Radboud Medical Center, in the town of Nijmegen, in the Netherlands. The bad news was that since they only did three or four Combidex MRIs a week, there was at least a six months' wait to get on the schedule.

I remembered the comforting words of Alfred E. Neuman of *Mad* magazine: "What, me worry?"

I filled in the forms and sent them off to the Netherlands.

By the following January, there was still no word from Nijmegen. I continued to track my PSA, eat less meat, get more exercise, and I kept on doing research for this book. It was embarrassing to realize how little I knew about my body. I learned, for example, that the seminal vesicles, a pair of tubular glands located behind and below the urinary bladder, secrete about 60% of the fluid that eventually becomes semen. What a rich cocktail of enzymes, proteins, fructose, vitamin C and flavins. Sounds like the original proto-typical baby formula. Only here's the bizarre part: normally, the seminal vesicles serve as the staging area from which the sperm begin their journey to the waiting egg. In my situation, however, they become a launching site from which cancer cells spread to the lymph system, and to the bones.

How's that for irony?

There was still no word from Nijmegen through February and March of 2007. Apparently Dr. Jelle Barentsz, who usually administers the Combidex MRI, was out on extended sick leave, and testing was proceeding at a snail's pace. For all I knew they might stop the Combidex testing entirely, which would leave thousands of guys like me in limbo.

Then one day Mark said, "You could still go for a knockout with IMRT. It's the best form of radiation as far as I'm concerned. You might want to check it out."

For "knockout," read "cure." Maybe it really was finally time.

I knew that IMRT—Intensity Modulated Radiation Therapy—was a significant improvement over the old forms of external beam radiation. And if it actually killed the cancer cells, suddenly the idea of having my prostate fried by electrons didn't seem quite so alarming, especially since getting onto the Combidex list was no sure thing, and the uncertainty was beginning to wear on my nerves. As four-letter words go, "cure" had a sweet ring to it.

Mark offered to call his friend, Lisa Chaiken, the chief radiation oncologist at the Santa Monica Treatment Center, a state-of-the-art facility for IMRT in Los Angeles. She was willing to see me right away for a consult.

A DAY AT THE RADIOACTIVE BEACH

Before going to see Dr. Chaiken, I checked out IMRT with Dr. Google. As Mark discussed earlier (see chapter 12), IMRT is a precisely targeted procedure that delivers high doses of radiation to the prostate and, when necessary, to the seminal vesicles and other surrounding tissue. The eight-to nine-week procedure significantly lowers the risk of tissue and organ damage. The big advantage of IMRT over regular external beam radiation is that you can shape the beam to the exact dimensions of the area you want to radiate. What's more, you can modulate the intensity within the beam itself (actually a variety of small independent beams) so that you curve the radiation dose around critical structures, such as the bladder or rectum, in order to protect them from damage, while maximizing the dose to the prostate gland and other target tissue. Instead of a solid beam of uniform intensity, you can achieve areas of high, medium and low dosage. Because of the complexity of the treatment plan, radiation oncologists employ special high-speed computers, treatment-planning software, diagnostic imaging and patient-positioning devices to plan treatments and control the radiation dosage during therapy.

Dr. Chaiken, a slender, handsome, dark-haired woman, was welcoming and generous with her time. When I had told her my history, she said, "When you were first diagnosed, IMRT wasn't available. With this new technology, the chance for a cure is substantially higher than with external beam radiation, and the likelihood of adverse side effects is dramatically less."

She introduced me to her IMRT colleagues, a group as impressive as a rocket science team. There was a medical physicist (a PhD with training in medical physics applications), a dosimetrist (who sets the radiation dosage), three therapists, and a radiation oncology nurse specialist. The nurse specialist, Janet Revell-Williams, told me she has been working in this field for twenty-two years. Obviously IMRT is by no means a pickup game of shooting hoops.

Dr. Chaiken showed me where they prepare the specially tailored, plastic body mold. "We make a mold for your lower back, hips and upper legs," she explained. "We choose an isocenter or reference point over the prostate for the field setup. We print three small tattoos on your belly to guarantee the same setup each day. We do a CAT scan and an MRI. We plan the radiation for all features by drawing in the computer the prostate, bladder, rectum, hips, penile bulb, lymph nodes and seminal vesicles. Then we prescribe the doses. Different sets of eyes look at everything. The team of the physician, physicist and dosimetrist determines the dose distributions. The chief tech does the setup session and makes sure the final plan is user friendly. Then, after any last adjustments, he puts all the data on a disc. After confirming the plan, we do a phantom run, using a water pool the shape of the pelvis as our target. Finally, a setup confirmation of the field is done with a BAT ultrasound."

The acronym BAT, she explained, stands for B-Mode Acquisition and Targeting through ultrasound. It indicates how the ultrasound is interpreted when rolled across the pelvis to measure the echo and to account for any movement of the prostate. According to Dr. Chaiken, "It ultrasounds externally, over the skin, the bladder, rectum, prostate, prostatic bed, and then pulls up the initial CT scans and MRIs that we use to plan the patient for radiation, and realigns the patient with that initial plan. It acquires the images and then targets them, making sure everything lines up before treatment. We do one reading before starting radiation treatment, and because the prostate actually *moves*, shifts its position from day to day, we do a new reading every day. Those daily readings determine how to shift the patient to be exactly lined up with real time anatomy."

Well *that* was thorough. I couldn't help thinking of the little girl who read a book on penguins and then wrote the author to say, "Dear Sir, Your book has told me rather more about penguins than I really care to know." Actually, the complexity and precision of the IMRT "event" was anything but boring. Still, what mattered most for me, since the cancer was already in the left seminal vesicle, was that IMRT covers both the prostate *and* the seminal vesicles.

We entered the radiation treatment room that housed the twelve-foot-tall linear accelerator. The walls were painted from floor to ceiling in tropical colors, with ocean scenes, frothy waves, sandy beach and palm trees. Dr. Chaiken smiled at me and said, "We try to make the place look like a day at the beach." But all I was thinking about was how they planned to shoot a mountain of energy at my pelvis from this giant ray gun, the muzzle of which would be situated barely two inches from my pecker.

Finally, Dr. Chaiken told me about what she called "the most dreaded complication," the possibility of permanent rectal burn, although with new techniques and equipment, she explained, the burn rate had dropped to less than 3%.

"This matter of rectal burn can't be ignored," she said. "Generally, however, rectal irritation is temporary, and can be relieved with medications. To have a long-lasting problem is very rare. So far we haven't seen it here."

That sounded reassuring until I checked out the possible side effects that came with that 3%: bleeding, pain, loss of rectal control and loss of rectal *sensation*, meaning, the inability to distinguish between gas, stool or liquid when you feel pressure. Gross! If you happen to fall into the 3%, you're screwed. Seems there is no known therapy that can effectively ameliorate the condition. The idea of rectal burn (also known as severe radiation proctitis and referred to by some docs as "hamburger ass"), however rare it may be, put my Refusenik-self on high alert and looking for the exit.

I thanked Dr. Chaiken and said I hoped we could meet again when I returned from the Netherlands.

As I was leaving, I noticed a sign on the wall: "Caution High Radiation Area," and a signal light in the form of a red glass balloon blinking over the treatment room door. It reminded me of the red warning light you see outside a sound stage when they're shooting. Only here the warning meant "Radioactive Procedure in Progress." Beyond that door, some guy was nestled into his own personal plastic womb, receiving one of forty-five treatments lasting about twenty minutes each. Total cost: approximately $40,000. Price of admission to the radioactive beach.*

After my meeting with Dr. Chaiken, I found myself brooding about my situation: *How long had the cancer been out of the capsule? What if I had already waited too long?* I'd had it with not knowing, and IMRT began to sound like a reasonable option despite the shadow cast by the 3% risk. The odds were favorable, the likelihood of a cure good. The more expert the team, the less risk, and Dr. Chaiken's team was undoubtedly among the best. I could actually see myself signing up for IMRT. However, if there was already lymphatic involvement, IMRT alone might be a massive waste of taxpayers' money. So once again, I found myself straddling the fence.

Then, on May 28, the day after my seventy-fifth birthday, I received an e-mail from St. Radboud Medical Center. A place had opened up in the Combidex MRI schedule on July 30. I called Jeanne, who was on the Greek island of Ikaria at the time, and told her the news.

The next day we bought our tickets to Amsterdam.

THE DUTCH CONNECTION

Jeanne and I arrived in the Netherlands on Friday, July 26. I had flown nonstop 5,700 miles from L.A. Jeanne had traveled by ferryboat from Ikaria to Athens, then by Olympic Airlines from Athens to Amsterdam. In seventy-two hours we would know if a gang of rogue cancer cells had set up housekeeping in my lymph glands.

It rained that night, a driving rain that pelted the windows of the houseboat where we were staying with our musician friend, Burton Greene. Lying in the dark, listening to my honey's calm breathing, my main feeling was one of gratitude for her love and support. Jeanne is a keen observer. From the moment when Jeff Harris found the dreaded lump, almost eighteen years ago, she had been at my side, weighing the options, giving me her perspective, accepting my decisions without flinching. I know she had buried much of her concern, not wanting to add her anxiety to my own. Rather than discussing the worst-case scenario, we sometimes took refuge in silence. As if merely talking about an ugly possibility gave it energy.

---

* With new technology (such as Varian's Rapid Arc treatment planning) that utilizes state-of-the-art linear accelerators with higher output of dose, treatment times are reduced to three to five minutes, depending on the extent of disease being treated. This makes the procedure much more comfortable for the patient. Moreover, the likelihood of internal organ movement during treatment is reduced, resulting in more accurate delivery of dose.

Neither of us had visited the Netherlands before, and we spent Saturday morning wandering in the dappled shade beside canals, through an endless thicket of bicycles, and weaving our way through a crowded street market. Beneath a flotilla of green umbrellas, the noisy outdoor bazaar was packed with stalls selling wines, wild mushrooms, Dutch cheeses, clogs, vintage clothing, stacks of 78 rpm records and volumes bound in cracked leather. Later we found our way to the magnificent house where Rembrandt had lived. Seeing the collection of Rembrandt's sketches had been Jeanne's lifelong dream—a dream finally realized thanks to the cancer, the unlikeliest of travel agents. It was an altogether lovely day, a bright shining stream flowing into an uncertain future.

On Sunday, we traveled by fast train to the 2,000-year-old town of Nijmegen. In 104 AD, the Emperor Trajan named the place *Ulpia Noviomagus Batavorum*, for short *Noviomagus*, ultimately rendered as *Nijmegen*. Charlemagne hung out there. And among other notables, Henrietta Pressburg, the mother of Karl Marx, was born there. Then, in 2005, Nijmegen became the Elba for the exiled Combidex.

Monday was another sunny, breezy day. We walked from our pension to the University Medical Center located on Geert Grooteplein and named for St. Radboud of Utrecht (850–917 AD; Feast Day, November 29). St. Radboud is almost the size of Cedars Sinai or Columbia Presbyterian. All the departments are numbered and color coded. Sunlight came slanting in through large windows as we followed the overhead signs in Dutch and stripes painted on the floor leading to the Radiology Section.

Dr. Noburu Takahashi, with his shock of black hair and big smile, looked like a teenager, certainly not someone old enough to be practicing medicine. He was standing in for Dr. Barentsz, who was still out with severe back problems. Patient and enthusiastic, Takahashi-san told us that the reason they performed so few Combidex MRI examinations per week was because of limited availability of the contrast agent and limited available time on the scanner. Furthermore, he explained, each evaluation took him at least one hour, plus another hour to complete his report. And he had numerous other duties.

Takahashi-san led me into a treatment room where I was hooked up to an IV drip for an infusion of the contrast agent. Once he had placed the needle in my vein, the procedure took about thirty minutes. There was no discomfort. Over the next twenty-four hours the nanoparticles of iron oxide would be picked up by the macrophages (from the Greek meaning "big eaters") and transported through my blood. I was told to return the following morning at 9:00 AM for the MRI. I had zero adverse reaction to the contrast agent. Piece of cake. And that night, I lay in bed picturing the nanoparticles circulating in my bloodstream, finding their way to *all* my healthy lymph nodes.

I have a photograph Jeanne snapped of me about to slide into the tunnel of the magnetic resonance machine. In the picture, I am wearing blue scrubs and am trussed up tight by a series of wide, white straps. I look like a 220-pound blue sausage in red socks.

I was in the machine for nearly an hour, and afterwards, Jeanne and I went to the cafeteria and had lunch. When we returned, Takahashi-san greeted us with a broad smile.

"All good," he said. "Lymph nodes all clear. Congratulations."

THE ROOTS OF THE TREE

Along with the good news, Takahashi-san gave me the stunning picture generated by magnetic resonance imaging. It looks like a forest of underground roots, twisted and contorted, tightly wrapped around each other; in structural anatomical terms, a magical tree that exists to handle blood flow.

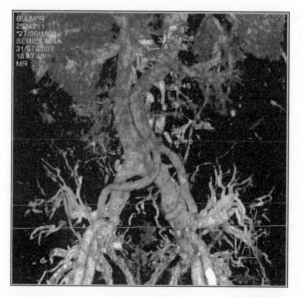

Image 3. Arteries and veins and cancer-free lymph node.

Image 3 shows a large artery and a large vein, and in the middle of the picture, you can see the abdominal aorta bifurcating or dividing into the left and right iliac arteries.

From my point of view, the most important elements in the picture are the numbered green structures—the periaortic lymph nodes scattered up and down the course of the aorta. *Green for cancer free.*

Healthy lymph nodes! What a blessing! With a huge weight removed from my mind, I resolved to stick with active surveillance, and Jeanne and I flew to Greece for a break.

And yet, grateful and relieved as I was, I was left with an uneasy feeling about the stunning difficulty and expense required to get an "All Clear!" for my lymph system. The Combidex procedure is low risk, better than 90% reliable and, as of 2010, far and away the best diagnostic test of its kind available anywhere. If it were available in the States, guys in my "at risk" position would be lining up around the block for the test.

I was puzzled about the failure of Combidex to make it past the FDA watchdogs. Since there's nothing else remotely like it, and since it does no harm, and since so many men are left in the dark and desperate to know about lymph gland involvement, why had the FDA trashed Combidex? I decided to find out.

THE DOCTOR'S VIEW

The ultimate question in cancer management is always the same: Has the cancer spread? Metastasized cancer is potentially life threatening. Cancer that stays home in the prostate is not. It's as simple as that. Yet, until Combidex, there has been no accurate test to detect small metastasis even though we know exactly where to look—in the lymph nodes. Sadly, here in the United States we are trying to answer the all-important lymph node question with an inadequate system that amounts to nothing more than sophisticated profiling. Take the PSA, the Gleason score, the biopsy findings, the grade, roll all the information together, and you have a *percentage estimate* for lymph node spread. We rely on *risk estimates* to guide treatment decisions by separating men into categories of *Low-, Intermediate-* and *High-Risk*. This methodology is fully elaborated in the next chapter and forms the basis for making important decisions about whether to operate, radiate or start TIP.

16.

DECIDING ON YOUR TREATMENT

And in the end, it's not the years in your life that count.
It's the life in your years.

—ABRAHAM LINCOLN

Up to this point we have been providing information about all the different options. Now is the time to *compare* treatments and decide which is best for you as an individual. With other cancers, the main issue is survival. With prostate cancer, we have a different priority. Real estate agents joke that the three most important considerations for selecting a property are location, location and location. For picking prostate cancer treatment, the three most important considerations are *quality of life, quality of life and quality of life*. Quality of life is the imperative because dying from properly diagnosed prostate cancer is unusual. Since long survival is the norm, anyone having to suffer damaging side effects will be burdened for many years.

Some may argue that excellent survival is not universal because men with *High-Risk* disease have increased cancer mortality. This is true, but only up to a certain point. For example, statistics from the Mayo Clinic published in the *Journal of Urology* in April 2008 show that only 2% of men with *Intermediate-Risk* and only 5% of men with *High-Risk* disease die from prostate cancer within ten years.[1] Therefore, even men with *High-Risk* disease need to think about quality of life.

The complex problem of comparing different treatments is more manageable if it can be broken down into smaller components. Prostate cancer is not a single illness. Therefore, treatment selection starts with separating men into *Low-, Intermediate-* and *High-Risk*. For men with *Low-Risk* prostate cancer the decision is simple: active surveillance. Active surveillance avoids the toxic side effects of immediate treatment without sacrificing the chance for cure or impairing long-term survival. Until a nontoxic treatment for prostate cancer is discovered, where quality of life is concerned, nothing compares to active surveillance. Conversely, with *Intermediate-Risk* or *High-Risk* disease many choices are available.

HIGH-RISK DISEASE

There are fewer options for *High-risk* disease so decision making is less complicated than with *Intermediate-Risk* disease. Randomized prospective studies in men with *High-Risk* disease show that radiation combined with TIP is superior to either radiation alone or TIP alone.[2,3,4] However, the optimal duration of TIP is controversial. A study published in the *New England Journal of Medicine* in June 2009 compared giving TIP for thirty months versus using TIP for only six months. The men treated for thirty months had better survival rates. However, no studies have tested continuing TIP for twelve to eighteen months to see if survival would be just as good as thirty months. This is a critical unanswered question because the longer TIP is continued the greater are the negative side effects.

Surgery for *High-Risk* disease is risky because positive margins are common (meaning that cancer is left behind after the operation) leading to further treatment with radiation and TIP, an undesirable triple whammy of treatments. Expert preoperative staging with color Doppler ultrasound or spectrographic endorectal MRI, though not perfect, makes a triple whammy less likely. Without expert preoperative evaluation, surgery for *High-Risk* disease is something of a crapshoot because there is a high chance that further therapy with radiation and TIP will be required.

INTERMEDIATE-RISK DISEASE

The decision-making process with *Intermediate-Risk* disease is the most complicated of all because men need to be educated about an extensive array of choices. Again, quality of life is the most important factor in the selection process. Therefore very careful attention must be paid to the long-term side effects of treatment. The remainder of this chapter will focus on those side effects. A number of scientific articles referenced at the end of this book have been published on this topic and reviewing them may be useful for those of you who want to delve deeper.[5,6,7,8,9,10]

To simplify the decision-making process, I recommend grouping the options of surgery, seeds and IMRT (termed "local treatments") on the one hand, and comparing them to TIP on the other. Local treatments affect only the prostate. TIP impacts the whole body. The advantage of local therapy is cure, whereas the advantage of TIP is being spared from permanent impotence, incontinence or rectal damage.

Side Effects of TIP

Blocking testosterone has wide-ranging side effects that fall into two groups: those preventable with a pill and those that are not so simple. First, the latter group, which includes side effects such as loss of libido, reduced muscle mass and weight gain.

Loss of Libido Libido is defined as sexual attraction. Libido is different from potency, which is defined as the ability to get an erection. With miracle drugs like Viagra, potency can exist without libido. Back in the 1990s we studied Viagra in a small group of twenty men on TIP. Nineteen reported back to us that they could perform sexually.[11] However, getting the study accomplished was a real chore. Time after time the study participants returned to our office with the sheepish excuse, "I forgot to take the Viagra." TIP had sapped all their interest in sex. To complete the study I had to resort to phoning them at home to remind them to take their pill. Their typical reaction was gracious. They seemed to understand the need to move the field of scientific endeavor forward. "Sure, Doc, I'll do it for you" was their joking reply.

I share this somewhat humorous experience because it illustrates how completely sexual desire is eradicated by TIP. Male libido is a pervasive part of a man's day-to-day mentality. Initially, men simply don't believe me when I warn them about TIP's effect on libido. But a few months after starting TIP, when the libido is gone, they come to the office with a wide-eyed look and confess, "When you told me about losing my libido, I thought it was impossible. I was convinced my sex drive was too strong to be eradicated by anything."

Loss of libido from TIP is very common but not quite universal. In my experience libido is completely lost in 90% of men over age seventy, 80% of men in their sixties and two-thirds of men in their fifties. Libido returns when testosterone recovers. However, even after testosterone recovery, about 25% of men over age sixty-five describe their libido as less intense than it was prior to starting TIP.

Loss of testosterone has another negative effect. Men normally have an average of three to five erections at night, but these nocturnal erections usually cease on TIP. The absence of this natural "nighttime exercise" can cause permanent shrinkage of a man's erection. To offset this we prescribe Viagra, Levitra or Cialis three times a week to maintain function.

Loss of Muscle Mass For years we counseled men that the main concerns with TIP are loss of libido and fatigue. Back in the 1990s some men on TIP would come to the office looking like limp dishrags. For unknown reasons, other men would appear just fine. This mystery was unraveled when for fitness reasons I started working out with weights. My new sideline led to conversations with some of my patients who were also weight lifting. Finally I made the connection. Those who were lifting weights almost never developed severe tiredness from TIP. In other words, their tiredness was directly related to muscle loss. A randomized prospective trial in Canada comparing quality of life in TIP-treated men with or without exercise has confirmed the importance of weight training on TIP.[12]

Weight Gain Loss of testosterone also slows body metabolism. Eating the same diet you have followed all your life can easily cause a weight gain of ten or twenty pounds. At the start of TIP it is wise to evaluate one's diet for excess fat and sugar and make the necessary changes.

Side Effects of TIP That Are Reversible with Medications

Low testosterone induces a variety of side effects that can be controlled with medications. However, minimizing the impact of TIP requires a willingness to use these medications consistently.

Hot Flashes Hot flashes occur in about two-thirds of men treated with TIP. They are severe enough to require treatment in about one out of five. The most effective treatment is estrogen. Eighty percent of men treated with an estrogen patch will have a dramatic reduction in the incidence and intensity of the hot flashes. Progesterone also works. One convenient option is a single injection of a medication called Depo-Provera.

Other medications are Effexor or Neurontin. Studies also show that acupuncture can be effective.[13]

Breast Growth If preventative measures are not used, breast enlargement occurs to some degree in about one-third of men. Femara, an estrogen-blocking pill, should be started at the first sign of breast tenderness or enlargement. Fully developed breast enlargement is only reversible with cosmetic surgery or liposuction.

Osteoporosis Prior to starting treatment men should obtain a baseline bone density test since TIP causes accelerated calcium loss from the bones similar to what postmenopausal women who lose their estrogen experience. Untreated bone loss can result in hip and spine fractures. Osteoporosis is preventable with bone-building medications such as Boniva or Actonel given as a once-a-month pill. These medications, along with vitamin D and calcium, should be started routinely when TIP is initiated. (See chapter 22 for more information on osteoporosis.)

Arthritis Joint pains, particularly in the hands but sometimes in other joints, are common with TIP though actual joint damage does not occur. The discomfort responds well to over-the-counter preparations like glucosamine, MSM, and super oxide dismutase (SOD). Typical nonsteroidal anti-inflammatory drugs like Motrin and Celebrex are also quite effective. The joint pains go away when TIP is stopped.

Mood Swings Men on TIP occasionally comment about becoming more emotional. For example, they may cry more easily at the movies. For some this is embarrassing. Others, like Ralph, enjoy it as a positive development. For men in the former situation, small doses of common antidepressant medication (such as Zoloft or Paxil) restore the intensity of feeling back to the normal range.

Conclusions Regarding TIP Side Effects

Taking TIP for a year is a considerable undertaking. After the treatment is stopped an additional three to four months are needed for the body to regenerate testosterone. Generally life reverts to normal as long as appropriate preventative measures are followed during treatment.

SURGERY VS. SEEDS VS. IMRT FOR MEN
WITH *INTERMEDIATE-RISK* DISEASE

Many patients with *Intermediate-Risk* prostate cancer conclude that with the local treatments such as radiation or surgery, quality of life will be better by curing the disease. Although these treatments eliminate the prostate gland and the cancer within, men need to consider the potential side effects in advance because they are often irreversible. Table 5 below lists the common long-term side effects and their frequency. The percentages listed are for a sixty-five-year-old man with good preexisting erectile function and a prostate that is not excessively enlarged.

Table 5:* Long-term Side Effects and Frequency

	Impotence	Incontinence	Urethritis	Stricture	Proctitis
Surgery	50%	8%**	-	5%	-
Seeds	35%	-	10%	1%	1%
IMRT	35%	-	2%	-	2-4%

* The percentages represent the results of top doctors throughout the U.S. The risk of side effects is much worse when less qualified doctors are performing the therapy and when men are older than sixty-five.

** The risk of incontinence is higher in men with a short membranous urethra less than 12mm long. Men contemplating surgery should have an endorectal MRI or color Doppler ultrasound prior to surgery to determine their anatomy.[14]

All the effects in the table are treatable. However, total reversal is usually not possible. Doctors define impotence as the inability to get an erection firm enough for penetration even though Viagra or a similar drug is being used. Impotence can be correctable with surgical placement of a penile implant. Studies indicate that satisfaction rates with implants are about 85% when the prosthesis is placed by an experienced surgeon.

Surgery that causes urinary incontinence persisting more than a year is generally permanent. Usually, but not always, incontinence can be helped with the surgical implantation of an artificial sphincter. Proper insertion requires considerable skill and should be performed only by experienced doctors who do it frequently.

Another risk of surgery is the problem of stricture, a type of scarring that blocks the flow of urine through the urethra. Until recently, corrective treatment consisted of forcing larger and larger probes up the penis to dilate the constricted area. However, studies now show that this often fractures the brittle scar tissue, causing incontinence. Urethral stricture is best managed with an operation performed at a center of excellence specializing in this proceedure.

Seed implants can induce urethritis, a radiation burn to the urinary passage through the prostate. The symptoms of severe urethritis are similar to those of a urinary tract infection and include burning pain, the need to urinate frequently, and an urgent and compelling need to urinate *right now*. These symptoms may respond partially to various medications. In the worst cases, urethritis from a seed implant can take up to two or three years to resolve.

IMRT can be associated with proctitis, a radiation burn of the rectum. Chronic proctitis is rare, but when it occurs, typically shows up a year or two after treatment. Its symptoms—pain, urgency, bleeding and fecal incontinence—can be ameliorated to some degree with cortisone enemas. Unfortunately, relief is almost always temporary.

All the potential long-term effects noted in the table can also occur on a short-term basis. In fact, right after surgery, the rate of impotence is 100%. If potency returns, it occurs slowly over many months. Severe symptoms of urethritis lasting for a couple of months occur in about two-thirds of men who undergo seed implants. Mild proctitis symptoms lasting a month or so occur in about half of men who are treated with IMRT.

More Advantages and Disadvantages of Surgery

Radical prostatectomy is a major operation not to be taken lightly. The mortality rate from surgery consistently averages about one death for every 200 operations.[16,17] Cancer is left behind after the surgery (a positive margin) on average 25% of the time.[18] The side effects of robotic surgery are not that different from the older, open procedure. Robotic surgery offers smaller scars and a shorter hospital stay. However, in experienced hands important factors like potency and positive surgical margins are thought to be identical to the older methods.

An additional risk of surgery is shrinkage of the penis. This side effect was denied by surgeons for many years but studies show that average loss is about half an inch.[15] An aggressive rehabilitation program using Viagra, vacuum pumps and injected prostaglandins may correct this to some degree. Dr. John Mulhall's book, *Sexual Function in the Prostate Cancer Patient*, should be required reading *before surgery* as some elements of the rehab process are more effective if started immediately after the operation.

When quoting potency rates, the definition of what constitutes an erection is often very loose. When potency is defined more precisely as having erections *identical* to before surgery, studies indicate that only 5–15%[19,20] of men have complete recovery. A few centers using the older, open procedure have arranged for independent verification of their potency rates by outside statisticians.[21] So far, robotic surgery centers have provided only *self-reported* statistics.

Microscopic examination of the surgically removed prostate gland provides additional information about the extent and grade of the cancer, which informs about the likelihood of future relapse. The removal of the prostate also creates a "clean slate" by removing all noncancerous PSA-producing prostate tissue. This simplifies PSA monitoring so that even slight elevations of PSA (above 0.07) accurately indicate relapsing cancer.

A Warning Concerning Surgery and Radiation

To this day patients are still being told the following outdated fallacy: "You can do radiation after surgery but surgery after radiation is very difficult." By saying this there is an implication that you will be somehow better off doing surgery since, that way, you have a second chance for cure with radiation. It's true that in the old days, prior to the advent of high-dose radiation, cancer often came back in the prostate gland after radiation treatment. This created a horrible dilemma because surgery after radiation is indeed much more technically difficult. Radiated body tissues heal poorly, leading to a much higher likelihood of surgical complications. However, modern high-dose radiation rarely results in isolated relapses in the prostate and these unusual cases can be treated with cryotherapy instead of surgery.

Rather than opting for surgery and using radiation as a backup, your real priority should be getting the job done right the first time.

More Advantages and Disadvantages of Seeds or IMRT

Permanent seed implantation is a relatively convenient treatment performed as a forty-five-minute outpatient procedure under spinal anesthesia. Unlike surgery, the onset of impotence, if it occurs, is usually delayed for several years. As mentioned above, the most common short-term effect of seed implantation is urethritis, which feels like a urinary tract infection. About two-thirds of patients experience some degree of urethritis and it typically lasts a couple of months. Patients who have enlarged prostate glands or pre-existing urinary symptoms from BPH are more prone to develop urethritis.

Patients who have seed implantation are at risk for developing a non-cancerous PSA rise one to four years after the implant, a phenomenon called the PSA "bump." Because a PSA increase can also signal a cancer recurrence, a bump engenders considerable anxiety. The only way a cancer recurrence can be distinguished from a bump is by checking PSA levels monthly. The PSA of men who are undergoing a bump seesaws up and down without any clear direction or trend. Conversely, a steady rise in PSA denotes a relapse. Some doctors unfamiliar with the bump mistakenly conclude that any sort of PSA elevation means that cancer is back.

Other than the need for daily travel to a specialized facility, IMRT has the lowest incidence of short-term side effects. Typically side effects, when they occur, are mild diarrhea, urethritis and fatigue for a couple of months. As with seeds, if impotence occurs, onset is usually delayed.

Advantages and Disadvantages of Cryotherapy

Skillfully administered cryotherapy to treat the whole prostate (rather than cryotherapy directed focally at the tumor as discussed in chapter 14) is effective at eradicating cancer. However, the popularity of whole-gland cryotherapy, compared to surgery or radiation, has been low due to the incidence of almost universal impotence. With surgery or radiation you have at least an even chance of maintaining erectile function. Therefore, whole-gland cryotherapy is reserved for men who have nothing to lose in this regard—the ones with preexisting impotence. Whole-gland cryotherapy is done in the hospital and requires a urinary catheter for a few days after the procedure. The risk of incontinence is about 5%. Very rarely, cryotherapy can cause an opening between the bladder and rectum, a fistula, which in some cases can be very difficult to correct.

FINAL THOUGHTS ABOUT DECIDING ON TREATMENT FOR *INTERMEDIATE-RISK* DISEASE

Soon after diagnosis men quickly discover that laypeople and professionals alike are bursting to share their opinion and they all seem to think they're experts. Run from these "experts"—doctors, friends or family—who preach simplistic answers with bombastic fervor. In the minds of these know-it-alls, all prostate cancer is life threatening. They have no idea of what they don't know. In my experience, the less people know, the more strongly they express their opinion.

To summarize as simply as possible, TIP is attractive because the side effects are reversible. However, although treatment with TIP buys you time, it does not result in a cure. On the other hand, local treatments are appealing because they often lead to cure—not a longer life—but a better quality of life by achieving closure. However, surgery and radiation involve betting all your chips on one roll of the dice. If no major side effects like impotence and incontinence occur, you win big. Conversely, when side effects occur, they can be permanent. So, bottom line, no treatment decision should be made until you have carefully weighed all the factors discussed above from a quality-of-life perspective.

In reality, there are no easy answers. Men usually reach a decision by finally deciding which treatments they *don't* want to do. What is left over, even though undesirable, is what they end up doing.

THE PATIENT'S VIEW

As my friend Bob Cooley put it, "Give it to me straight, Doc. And in eighth-grade English, just to be safe."

As Mark has said, "Deciding on the best treatment requires disciplined thinking as it relates to risk category." So if you're at the deciding stage, take a deep breath or take a shot of Jack Daniel's, read this chapter several times, and then decide what to do.

If you already know you have *Low-Risk* prostate cancer, you can safely defer making a decision, and stick with active surveillance. Get regular checkups. And if you have questions, talk to your primary care physician, your urologist or, if you have one, your oncologist.

17.

ANATOMY OF AN ASSISTED SUICIDE

The Oncologic Drugs Advisory Committee (ODAC) of the FDA voted
15 to 4 to not recommend approval of the proposed indication for
Combidex . . . The committee cited insufficient clinical data to support
a broad indication for use of Combidex to differentiate metastatic from
non-metastatic lymph nodes across all cancer types.

—FDA REPORT OF THE ODAC MEETING OF MARCH 3, 2005

Fired up by my experience with Takahashi-san, I was determined to find
out why the FDA had rejected Combidex back in 2005. Why is there just
one place in the world where you can get the Combidex MRI to find out
if the cancer has spread to your lymph nodes?

The obvious source was the CEO of Advanced Magnetics, Jerome
Goldstein. The problem was that Goldstein had retired in 2007. When I
spoke with the headquarters of Advanced Magnetics in Cambridge, Massachusetts, and asked how to reach Mr. Goldstein, they told me to send
an e-mail to their office and it would be forwarded. Not the approach I
wanted to take.

So I went into sleuth mode. If I were a CEO for a Cambridge company, I doubt that I would live in Cambridge. Why not? Assumption:
Goldstein probably plays golf, and there is no decent golf course in the
neighborhood. Where then? My freshman year in college, I dated a
young woman whose father, Luther Grimes, managed an ancient and
honorable golf club, The Country Club in Brookline. So I googled "Jerome Goldstein, Brookline, Massachusetts," and found a single listing,
but no data on his work history. Then I had another thought: try "Politi-
cal Contributions." Campaign contributions and donations are public
record and often easy to track. So back to Dr. Google. Again, I found
one Jerome Goldstein, with donation amounts listed year by year *and* living in Brookline. For Occupation: Retired. However, since I knew he'd

been with the company at the time of the 2005 FDA hearing, I scrolled back down the years to the "Presidential Elections of 2004." And there it was: a donation of $4,000 by Jerome Goldstein, *President of Advanced Magnetics*. Bingo!

Goldstein's telephone number was listed in the phone book. He answered on the second ring, and when I introduced myself he sounded wary. To reassure him that this wasn't some crank call, I ran a short list of Blum credentials: Andover, Harvard, cowriting a book with a prostate oncologist, just returned from Nijmegen.

The fact that I had gone to Holland for the Combidex MRI got his attention.

"So what do you want to know?" Goldstein asked.

"What went wrong? Why did the FDA reject Combidex? And can I quote you?"

"I'm retired now," Goldstein said in a gruff voice. "So I suppose you can quote me. Some of the blame was ours. Our application was too broad. We should have gone for disease specificity. But that's only part of it. The FDA bureaucrats in ODAC were also to blame. ODAC—that's the Oncologic Drugs Advisory Committee—has total control over the life and death of every new application. And because of ODAC's decision, patients are dying and suffering needlessly."

What Goldstein meant when he said their "application was too broad" and that they "should have gone for disease specificity" was that instead of specifying Combidex as a contrast agent for establishing lymph node involvement in *one* type of cancer—prostate cancer—Advanced Magnetics had tried to broaden its application to cover *all* cancers. However, their research and trials had focused only on prostate cancer. They didn't have sufficient numbers to show the efficacy of Combidex for other cancers. So going for what is known as a broader "indication" (in this case a general lymph node indication) was not a smart move.

When I asked Goldstein what happened at the ODAC meeting, he didn't hesitate. "The chairwoman that day terminated the meeting before the Committee got to questions of a narrower indication. The broader indication, that was, well, I'll call it Step One on the agenda. But when we got to the end of Step One, she called for a vote. We never got to address questions Two, Three and Four that dealt with more limited indications. She just cut off the debate. It was a farce."

"That really sucks."

"Oh, there's more," Goldstein said. "We brought in expert witnesses to tell how beneficial Combidex MRI had been. People like Tom Brady, who is head of Imaging Research at Mass General. He paid his own way down to Maryland to make a plea for approval. Once it was approved, it could be used off label.'"

"Off label" is the other term, along with "indication," that plays a significant role in the Combidex story. Once a drug is approved for any single indication, it is legal for doctors to use it "off label," meaning, wherever, in their judgment, it is useful.

I asked Goldstein if it was possible to obtain a transcript of the ODAC meeting, and he told me that their meetings were a matter of public record.

Then, in a low angry growl, he said, "Nobody should ever die from this disease. It's a crime."

I thanked him and said I would get back to him after I did my homework. I was about to hang up, when he said, "You know I have prostate cancer. I was diagnosed two years ago. Gleason 6. My internist said I should do surgery or put seeds in."

"So what did you do?"

"Nothing."

"Nothing?"

"Well, not exactly nothing. I bought a new putter."

ODAC: THE FDA'S FIRING SQUAD

Although the transcripts of FDA meetings are a matter of record, they are not that easy to find. What's more, they are not indexed so you have to dig. When I finally read the minutes and watched a video of the March 3, 2005 ODAC meeting, it was painfully obvious that there was plenty of blame to go around. But the way Combidex—NDA Application 21-115—went down, really pissed me off.

The meeting took place at the Hilton Hotel in Gaithersburg, Maryland, in the Grand Ballroom, a space of almost 3,900 square feet. There were TV cameras facing a U-shaped table where the Voting Committee sat, with the chairperson seated at the head of the table. At a second U-shaped table facing it, sat the Advanced Magnetics team, a group from Mass General and a number of other witnesses. Beyond that was the public area with space for about four hundred. Coffee and pastries were provided for the experts and the Voting Committee.

The ODAC Committee is generally made up of oncologists from various fields including hematology and radiation oncology, as well as consumer and patient representatives. The Chairperson that day, Silvana Martino, DO, opened the meeting and then turned it over to George Mills, MD, the FDA Division Director for Medical Imaging and expert on drug safety.

Here's how Mills began: "The Agency is asked to consider an indication specifically for differentiating metastatic from non-metastatic lymph nodes"—and then came the first red flag—*"with little restriction on the cancer type, clinical staging, and whether the patients have been properly treated"* (my italics).

Mills made it clear that this was the second review cycle, meaning Combidex had failed to pass on the first round. He then said that Advanced Magnetics had been instructed to conduct additional studies to address issues related to "inconsistent efficacy results," to provide "clearer identification for the conditions of use for Combidex" and to address "safety issues related to Combidex-induced hypersensitivity reactions."

Mills also pointed out that Advanced Magnetics planned to use data already submitted, and to rely heavily on a study published in the June 19, 2003 *New England Journal of Medicine*. The article was entitled, "Noninvasive Detection of Clinically Occult Lymph-Node Metastases in Prostate Cancer." Given the prominence of its eight international authors and the prestigious nature of the *NEJM*, its conclusion—that "high-resolution MRI with magnetic nanoparticles allows the detection of small and otherwise undetectable lymph-node metastases in patients with prostate cancer"—represented powerful support for Combidex.

However, the following speaker, Dr. Zili Li, Medical Team Leader with the Division of Medical Imaging and Radiopharmaceutical Drug Products at the FDA, brought up a problem. Dr. Li claimed that after repeated requests, Advanced Magnetics had failed to provide the FDA with the original source document for the *NEJM* article. Therefore the Agency could not conclude that the study was conducted in compliance with the federal regulations pertaining to a new drug application or that it qualified as an adequate and well-controlled study.

When I next spoke with Jerome Goldstein about the FDA's judgment call on the *NEJM* article, he gave me the background. Advanced Magnetics had not ignored the FDA's requests. They had pushed hard to obtain the original source document, only it turned out that, since the article's publication, the *NEJM* had moved offices three times. In the repeated packing and unpacking, apparently the source document was lost. However, according to Goldstein, the FDA had twisted the facts to indicate that Advanced Magnetics had failed to comply with their repeated requests.

Dr. Li also drew attention to Advanced Magnetics' "broad indication." He pointed out that, if FDA approved, Combidex could be "used for almost all cancers regardless of type, size, clinical stage, whether the patient had been previously treated with drug, biologic, radiation, or surgery." He then proceeded to address the agency's concerns for such a broad indication "given the level of efficacy and safety observed from clinical trials."

What I learned next may have been what sealed Advanced Magnetics' fate. Apparently one of their early test subjects had died. They gave the guy an injection of Combidex and he went into anaphylactic shock. The fact that this single death had occurred a decade earlier, and had resulted in an immediate shift in method of delivery—from injection, to dilution of the contrast agent in saline and use of slow infusion—did not reassure the FDA.

Dr. Li expressed another major concern, which was that Advanced Magnetics did not have appropriate personnel available to cope with such an emergency, and that by the time the EMT arrived and delivered CPR and epinephrine, it was too late: the man died at the hospital thirty-five minutes later. To make matters worse, Dr. Li said that the FDA did not consider dilution and slow infusion as entirely risk free, and claimed that there was some disparity between U.S. and European test procedures. Advanced Magnetics, however, pointed out that the vast majority of test subjects had only very minor and transient adverse (mainly allergic) reactions and that only four out of 1,236 patients had experienced a more serious adverse reaction. With the new method of administration, there had been no further deaths and no serious side effects.

I later learned from the Combidex records that the man who had died was so eager to participate in the trials that he failed to disclose his allergic condition, or that he had gone into anaphylactic shock on other occasions.

THE VIEW FROM ADVANCED MAGNETICS

I wanted to confirm the information in the ODAC transcript, so I spoke with one of the most knowledgeable former staff members at Advanced Magnetics who had attended the meeting—I'll call him Olof Bergen, MD. Here's how Dr. Bergen explained things.

"Advisory Committee Meetings are always a crapshoot. But that group was unusual. When we started our product development, there was an active FDA Medical Imaging Advisory Committee. But the FDA disbanded that Committee to save money, so our case went to ODAC. I was nervous about ODAC. Still, we thought their cancer specialists would see the advantages of Combidex. So I was totally unprepared for the outcome of the vote."

"How do you account for the rejection?"

"The FDA, in their presentation to ODAC, broke our proposal down by particular type of cancer, even though throughout our development of Combidex the FDA had *never* asked us to do that. We got twenty pages of instructions, which we followed precisely. They never told us we needed sufficient numbers in *each* type of cancer. The FDA-approved trial was designed on the premise that lymph nodes, wherever they are in the body, work the same way. They never told us we needed to do a statistical breakdown and show statistical significance by cancer type. And yet they presented the case to ODAC as if they had asked for all that, and we had failed to comply.

"And another thing," Dr. Bergen continued, "it's essential, when you're preparing to present, that you work with the same FDA people. Well, the medical reviewer who made the presentation to ODAC was not the medical reviewer who had reviewed the product during its ten-year development. That was Bob Yaes, a radiologist, a no-nonsense guy who had been difficult and critical of Combidex during the development process. But I met with him before the ODAC meeting, and he told me he had finally understood the benefit of the contrast agent and that he was recommending approval. Then at the last minute, they replaced him with Dr. Li, who had not been involved in the development phase at all. So we had no proof of what they had originally asked and not asked. And Li was not the only strange face. *All* of the players had changed. Not one of the people who had been involved in the development of Combidex was there that day.

Not one. In retrospect, we should never have allowed them to get away with that."

Dr. Bergen also told me about a fundamental problem with imaging substances. Contrast agents are regulated just like drugs: the same standards apply for a contrast agent as for an antibiotic used to treat a life-threatening infection. Apparently it takes an act of Congress to get contrast agents regulated differently from drugs and so far that hasn't happened. But it's obvious that there need to be different rules for approving imaging agents. "Just another disgrace," Dr. Bergen said. "Add it to the list."

MONEY MATTERS AND VIOXX: THE GHOST AT THE BANQUET

After interviewing several staff members at Advanced Magnetics, I became very aware of the financial reality. Contrast agents are not economically viable. They are subjected to all the same requirements as a drug, they can cost over $100 million to develop, and the likelihood of FDA approval is increased by having a narrow indication. But here's the irony: the narrower the indication, the less chance the company will ever recoup its money.

Advanced Magnetics did one major study with Combidex, plus several supporting studies, and according to staff members they had FDA approval for that approach. If they had done individual, well-controlled studies for breast cancer, bladder cancer, cervical cancer, lung cancer, liver cancer et cetera, the cost would have been totally prohibitive.

"You can't afford to do it," Dr. Bergen told me, "and the FDA people know that. Too broad an application? What a crock! A normal lymph node for somebody with breast cancer is no different than a normal lymph node for somebody with prostate cancer. Combidex is taken up *only* in normal tissue. If the tissue's not normal, the contrast agent is not taken up, and you know there's cancer."

So while it would appear that applying for a broad application not only made medical sense, it was the only hope Advanced Magnetics had of getting their money back. However, here's how it works: you get FDA approval for *one indication*, and then you go off label, meaning use it for other cancers at your discretion.

Which brings me to Vioxx, the ghost at the banquet.

Vioxx (rofecoxib) is a nonsteroidal anti-inflammatory drug to treat osteoarthritis, acute pain conditions and dysmenorrhea. It was approved as safe and effective by the FDA on May 20, 1999, and was marketed under the brand names of Vioxx, Ceoxx, and Ceeoxx. Worldwide, over eighty million people were prescribed rofecoxib. Then, on September 30, 2004, rofecoxib was withdrawn from the market because of an increased risk of heart attack and stroke.

"You have to consider the mood at that meeting," Dr. Bergen explained. "Vioxx had been having problems and was voluntarily withdrawn from the market because of safety issues, but not before Merck sales had passed $2.5 billion. Then, less than *two weeks* before Combidex came before ODAC, Merck announced that the return of Vioxx to the American market was 'uncertain.' The anxiety in the room was palpable. The focus was totally on safety. From what I've seen over the years, the FDA people don't regard imaging probes as important, so they consider any risk at all to be unacceptable. And frankly, the safety that concerns them is their own. No one at the FDA ever got a promotion for approving a drug. And if a drug you approve later turns out to have problems, there goes your career. So, yes, the recall of Vioxx had poisoned the atmosphere at that meeting at the Gaithersburg Hilton."

It didn't help the case for Advanced Magnetics when a veteran FDA researcher warned that "a profound regulatory failure in evaluating Vioxx could easily be repeated with other drugs." So it would seem highly plausible that even before Advanced Magnetics presented their case, the fix was in. The FDA had decided to make certain that Combidex would be regarded by the ODAC voting members as unsafe. Combidex was rejected by a vote of 15 to 4.

In one day, Advanced Magnetics stock dropped over 50%, and Combidex was dead in the United States. Ten years of research, Stage Three testing completed, thousands of hours and over $150 million lavished on a project to produce a test that has no equal, is 90% reliable, produces minimal side effects and is desperately needed—all that down the drain.

THE MYSTERY OF NANOPARTICLES

Before starting to write this chapter, I probably talked to a dozen or more people who were at that ODAC meeting. I found that a number of the participants could barely remember the event. No blame. It was too long ago. Others were still incensed that Combidex had been trashed.

One of the participants, a voting member whom I interviewed, was wary, somehow uneasy. Finally, after a few jars of *sake*, I learned why, and it wasn't anything that had surfaced in the testimony at the meeting. His vote against approval of Combidex resulted from his concern about the possible future consequences of a new technology—the small coated super-paramagnetic iron oxide nanoparticles.

And yet, as we talked, I realized that he considered Combidex extremely valuable. I said I didn't understand the reason for his "No" vote. Was there, I asked, something I was missing?

He shrugged. "For me, it's a safety issue."

"Are you thinking of the test subject who died? That was years ago."

"No, not that. But I will say, the surest way to kill someone in anaphylactic shock is to call 9-1-1. The patient had cardiovascular disease. If he'd been given oxygen immediately, and fluids to increase the blood pressure, he'd have been okay."

"You said that for you it was a safety issue. What did you mean by that?"

We each had another *sake*. And another. Silence. He seemed to be trying to come to a decision. Finally, he said, "You want to know how I feel? I'll tell you. But you can't use my name. Agreed?"

"Agreed."

"The whole business of nanoparticles makes me nervous, all right? These are *metal* particles. They conduct electricity. They interact with ions. They behave biologically in ways we can't predict. The claim is that they're taken out by the macrophages, that they're cleared from the blood within five days. Well, we don't know that for sure."

"But that's the science," I said.

"Not good enough. We need to follow patients who've gotten this contrast agent and see how they're doing five years, ten years out. We don't have the data. And, yes, that scares me. I can't speak for anyone else. Like it or lump it. That's why I voted how I voted."

I felt like I was down the rabbit hole with a possibly Mad Hatter. I said, "What about the guys who are at risk right now? Guys who need to know *now* if there's lymphatic involvement? They haven't got ten years or five years. If it's an aggressive cancer, they may not have five *months* unless they get immediate treatment."

"Yeah, well, that's a bitch."

We weren't getting anywhere. So I switched direction.

"Let's say, for the sake of argument, that the benefits outweigh the risks. What about compassionate use here in the U.S.?* Isn't that a standard provision with non-approved drugs?"

"Sure, you can go for compassionate use. But it's a big deal just to start the process. With Combidex, you'd have to find someone who's trained to interpret the results, someone who'll take time out of a busy practice to administer it. And even if you do find that someone, *and* you get permission from the FDA, then you have to get the contrast agent from Advanced Magnetics, and, well, they've moved on to other things. Anyway, that's the least of it. If you're right about the numbers—it's not just two or three guys—if it's really hundreds, have you thought of the paperwork involved? Compassionate use applies only on a case-by-case basis. You need the go-ahead from the FDA for *every single one of the subjects* . . . And I still have my concerns about the safety of the technology."

Realistic or not, there it was, one committee member's reasons for voting against approval. If the microparticles of iron *did* lodge in the walls of the heart or in a coronary artery, I suppose it's conceivable that they might precipitate clotting and cause a cardiac event. However, the original Combidex death was a guy who died of anaphylactic shock, not a heart attack.

A FLY-OVER BY THE LIBRARY ANGEL

After that interview, the matter of nanoparticles continued to haunt me. Then one day it occurred to me to talk with my friend, author Michael Crichton, who was also an MD, about the ODAC meeting. I knew Michael had been sick. But I also knew I could count on him for an informed opinion about whether the possibility of iron oxide nanoparticles lodging in the walls of the heart was a matter of real concern or total nonsense. So I called and left a message for him at his office.

I never got to ask Michael about his views on nanoparticles. On the night of November 5, 2008, I happened to turn on the *Charlie Rose* show, and there he was. It was the rebroadcast of an old interview. That was how I learned of Michael's death.

---

* Compassionate use: the term used in the U.S. for a means of providing experimental therapeutic products prior to final FDA approval for use in humans. This procedure is available only to very sick individuals who have run out of approved treatment options.

Then something strange happened. Have you ever heard of "the Library Angel"? You're looking for a particular book in a huge secondhand store, and *Shazam!* there it is on a cart, right in front of you. That's the Library Angel in action. I credit the Angel for bringing Jeanne and me together. Jeanne was in Annapolis twenty-eight years ago, looking for something in a bookstore when, as she puts it, *"The Book of Runes* [a work of mine] fell off the shelf into my hands." Jeanne eventually ended up writing to me. I liked her handwriting. I wrote back . . . The Library Angel as marriage broker.

You may find what I am about to report hard to believe, but I swear on a stack of Bibles that it's precisely what took place. I was sitting in the lobby of the Hotel Luxe on Sunset Boulevard, waiting for my friends, Naoyuki and Ayako, who were still in their room packing. I was editing a draft of this chapter, up through the end of the ODAC meeting and wondering whether to include my informant's anxiety about nanotechnology. The décor of the Luxe lobby was Bel Air expensive and glossy chic: white couches, tall mirrors, giant floral arrangements. And next to the couch where I was sitting, just beside my right shoulder, was a floor to ceiling bookshelf stocked with a collection of books, mostly upright, some stacked in flat piles of two or three, and every book covered in a plain white wrapper. A ghost library. I had no notion of the authors or titles. For all I knew, the "books" were blocks of wood or Styrofoam—a reasonable double-blind situation for what followed.

As I sat there thinking about the exile of Combidex to Holland, I reached up and pulled a book off the shelf. It *was* a real book, and when I removed the white jacket, there were the author's initials stamped on the cover: *MC,* as in "Michael Crichton." There were hundreds of books on those shelves. Figure the odds.

The book was Michael's novel, *Prey.* I'd read *Prey* when it came out in 2002, but I only remembered it vaguely. I started reading the Introduction. On page *xii,* I came across this passage:

Sometime in the twenty-first century, our self-deluded recklessness will collide with our growing technological power. One area where this will occur is in the meeting point of nanotechnology, biotechnology, and computer technology . . . Nanotechnology, the newest of these three technologies and in some ways the most radical . . . will provide everything from miniaturized computer components to new cancer treatments to new weapons of war.

I spent the next half hour eagerly leafing through Michael's book, checking for any further references to nanotechnology. Finally, on page 255 and continuing over to the next page, I found this:

> Nano-particles are small enough to get places nobody's ever had to worry about before. They can get into the synapses between neurons. They can get into the cytoplasm of cardiac cells. They can get into cell nuclei. They're small enough to go anywhere inside the body.

I kept reading and rereading the two passages. I couldn't get beyond those nine words: *They can get into the cytoplasm of cardiac cells . . .* Was that just Michael, at his intuitive best, writing fiction? Or was my anonymous informant's concern about the risks of nanotechnology realistic? Or was the Library Angel messing with my head? Time will tell. But thank you, old friend, for that nudge and a wink from the other side.

Over the following days, I found myself remembering a bit of verse from my childhood, one of those cautionary jingles that parents of my generation were so fond of repeating, I suppose because they emphasize the importance of paying attention to the little things in life. It goes like this:

> *For want of a nail, the shoe was lost*
> *For want of a shoe, the horse was lost*
> *For want of a horse, the rider was lost*
> *For want of a rider, the battle was lost*
> *For want a battle, the war was lost*
> *And all for the want of a horseshoe nail.*

In the end, for me at least, the fate of Combidex was cause for long thoughts. What an odd mix of events. An unnecessary death. The shadow cast by the ghost of Vioxx. A Committee Chairperson who ended a meeting prematurely. One man's refusal to trust a new technology. For want of such horseshoe nails, battles are lost.

A defeat? For sure, but as for this war, it's anything but over.

Dispatch from the front: A new therapeutic agent called Feraheme (feru-moxytol), produced by Advanced Magnetics (AMAG Pharmaceuticals), has been granted FDA approval for intravenous use as an iron replacement therapy for iron deficient anemia in adult patients with chronic kidney disease. Testing of ferumoxytol to replace Combidex as a contrast agent is now under way at Nijmegen Medical Center in the Netherlands.

THE DOCTOR'S VIEW

Ever since my entry into the field of medical oncology twenty years ago, there has been one overriding and unchanging wet blanket impeding medical progress—the FDA. Unfortunately, the story of how the FDA has blocked Combidex here in the United States is typical of numerous effective treatments that have been kept off the market.

Ralph's chapter explaining the Combidex fiasco illustrates how capricious the approval process can be when you have bureaucrats whose main interest is avoiding criticism for their missteps, rather than concern for the cancer patients who are dying because they are blocked from access to a lifesaving technology.

18.

THE INSULIN CONNECTION

Prostate cancer, depending on how it acts, can be compared to a tortoise, a hare, or a bird. The tortoise moves slowly—so slowly that you may not even bother to treat it.

—PAUL LANGE, MD

Men on active surveillance want to delay treatment as long as they can, as long as it's safe to do so. Ideally they would like to be able to monitor the situation indefinitely. The natural question then becomes, "If I'm going to be doing this for a long time, what lifestyle changes can inhibit cancer growth? What can I do to minimize the chance my small prostate cancer will progress?" In chapter 20 I discussed the supplements that are considered to be helpful. In this chapter I delve more deeply into the mechanisms that are thought to explain why a change in diet is so important.

Until recently, no one connected insulin to cancer growth. Speak of "lack of insulin," and everyone immediately thinks of diabetes. Now, however, researchers have arrived at two striking new realizations: first, that insulin deficiency inhibits the development of cancer, and even more significant, excess insulin in the blood acts as high-octane fuel for cancer growth.

The connection between high insulin blood levels and cancer growth came to my attention thanks to patients who adopted rigorous diets as their primary means for treating their cancer.

In December 2001, Thomas Mueller, a Los Angeles attorney, learned he had prostate cancer. He was only forty-five and newly married. Thomas's cancer was of the *Intermediate-Risk* variety. What made his situation particularly alarming, however, was his awareness that the common treatments—surgery and radiation—frequently cause impotence. "I couldn't take that risk," he said. "I had to find another way."

THE MACROBIOTIC APPROACH

Thomas is of medium height and slight build, with close-cropped, wavy blond hair. He is soft spoken yet intense, with a self-deprecating, wry sense of humor. An intelligent and disciplined researcher, he quickly became knowledgeable about prostate cancer. But he had a complicated history with cancer—a close call with melanoma when he was still in his twenties. "Having two cancers by age forty-five convinced me," he said, "that a serious change in lifestyle was necessary." With the guidance of his wife, who happened to be a teacher of macrobiotics, Thomas decided to undertake a strict program of diet combined with exercise to manage his cancer.

He began his macrobiotic regime immediately, and in three months his weight plummeted from 157 to 122. At that point he was beyond lean. He was also exercising intensely, including running a marathon. "At the end of that ordeal," he reported, "I was so hypoglycemic that I was hallucinating. I definitely don't recommend marathons on such a stringent diet." Over that same period his PSA dropped from 4.0 down to 1.5, an encouraging sign that his cancer was being held in check.

Reliance on macrobiotic diet and lifestyle as a form of treatment is not new. In the 1920s, Yukikazu Sakurazawa came to Paris from Japan. He took the name "George Ohsawa," and called his teaching "macrobiotics." Michio Kushi brought Ohsawa's work to the United States in 1949.[1,2] The basis of Ohsawa's philosophy was a belief that returning to the diet common in agrarian cultures, a diet followed throughout most of human history, could both prevent and counteract disease.

Thomas's "healing version" of the diet, tailored specifically for cancer patients, was particularly restrictive, consisting mainly of whole grains and vegetables. Staples included miso soup, brown rice, lentils and "sea vegetables" like nori and kelp. Strictly forbidden were all sugars, fats, meats, dairy, oils (with some allowance for cooking) and even most fruits. Processed foods like breads and pasta were also scrupulously avoided. Clearly this rigorous diet is not for the faint of heart. Moreover, proponents of a macrobiotic diet believe that the healing process is enhanced by each individual's involvement in preparing their own food—the antithesis of our prepackaged, microwave culture. The macrobiotic preference is always for food that is in season and locally grown. "The time for food gathering and preparation was so demanding," Thomas told me, "that I resigned from my law firm and committed all my energy to healing myself."

There is increasing medical evidence to support the effectiveness of diet in counteracting prostate cancer. Dr. Dean Ornish, of cardiac diet fame, has now moved boldly into the arena of diet therapy for treating prostate cancer. In the September 2005 issue of the *Journal of Urology*, Ornish published the results of a study that tested the effectiveness of an intensive dietary and lifestyle program. This program consisted of a vegan diet (vegetarian, non-dairy) supplemented with antioxidants such as lycopene, selenium and vitamin E. The program also called for moderate aerobic exercise and the use of stress management techniques. Ornish studied ninety-three men who, like Thomas, had chosen to avoid conventional invasive treatment for their prostate cancer. Half of these men were randomly allocated to the Ornish diet program while the remainder served as a nontreated comparison group. After twelve months, the men on the program had achieved a statistically significant reduction in their PSA levels.[3]

When Ornish did additional laboratory studies on the blood of his participants, the results were dramatic. Extracting serum from the men in both groups, he fed it to prostate cancer cells kept alive in Petri dishes. The cancer cells that were fed serum from men *not* on the Ornish program *grew eight times faster* than those cells receiving serum from men who were on the program.

HOW CANCER IS FUELED

Impressive as these results are, Ornish's article did not offer a theory that would explain why the program works. A review of Thomas's medical history, however, provided a clue. Whenever Thomas came into our office, even if it was after eating, his serum blood sugar was in the seventies, an unusually low value. Blood sugars in most patients, when checked after a meal, run as high as 120 to 150. It seemed logical to me that there could be a direct connection between low blood sugar levels and retarded cancer growth.

Actually, it is not surprising that suppressed blood sugar (glucose) levels could have a major impact on cancer growth. Glucose functions like gasoline, fueling all the cells in the body. Cancer cells are especially greedy for sugar because growing cells have even greater energy needs. This fact is dramatically illustrated by a frequently used scanning technology for detecting cancer throughout the body known as Positron Emission Tomography, or PET. The PET scan uses radioactive sugar injected into the bloodstream to locate tumors throughout the body. The uptake of glucose into the cancer cells occurs so swiftly that the cancer cells light up within ten minutes of the injection.

There is an additional reason that cancer cells require vastly more glucose to survive and proliferate than normal cells. This is because cancer cells run on a primitive and inefficient energy metabolism called anaerobic glycolysis that burns sugar without oxygen. Normal cellular aerobic glycolysis, the type of metabolism that uses oxygen, extracts eight times more energy from each glucose molecule. In other words, cancer cells are extraordinarily inefficient. They must absorb much larger amounts of glucose from the blood than normal cells.

INSULIN: THE REAL VILLAIN

All this would seem to indicate that blood glucose levels are the driving force in cancer growth. But it fails to explain the fact that diabetics—men with chronically high blood sugar—have *less* prostate cancer than men who are not diabetic.[4] Why would this be? *Because diabetes is a disease of insulin deficiency.* Insulin is manufactured and stored in the pancreas. Release of insulin into the blood occurs *in response to high glucose levels.* As blood sugar levels rise, insulin release accelerates. All the cells in the body, including cancer cells, require insulin to take glucose from the blood and absorb it. They can't absorb sugar without insulin to facilitate uptake.

The connection between diet and cancer, therefore, appears to hinge only indirectly on blood sugar levels. It is not high blood sugar per se, but rather the high level of insulin *triggered* by high blood sugar that stimulates rapid cancer growth. To confirm this, several studies report a connection between insulin and prostate cancer. Two of these studies demonstrate that high insulin levels are connected with a higher incidence of prostate cancer.[5,6] A third study has reported that increased insulin levels are associated with the development of more aggressive prostate cancer.[7] All of this supports the conclusion that *insulin itself, much more than glucose, is driving prostate cancer.*

It is not surprising that insulin incites cancer growth. Insulin is a type of growth hormone. In fact, the active ingredient in growth hormone is a biochemical structure so similar to insulin that it is called "insulin-like growth factor" or IGF-1. (Like insulin, IGF-1 has also been correlated with an increased incidence of prostate cancer.)

With such compelling evidence that insulin suppression is vital for controlling cancer, the real question is how to reduce insulin. At the present time, diet is the most effective method for controlling insulin levels. The basic dietary approach to minimizing insulin demand has been worked out for the treatment of diabetics in what is termed a low-glycemic index diet. The glycemic index (GI) ranks different foods on a scale from 0 to 100 according to the rapidity with which they raise blood sugar levels. High-glycemic foods result in more rapid increases in blood glucose levels than low-glycemic foods. A glycemic index below 55 is considered low. Levels above 70 are considered high. Examples of high-glycemic foods are potatoes (76) and bread (73). Examples of low-glycemic foods are nuts (22), lentils (29), raw apples (38) and brown rice (55). White rice is intermediate with a glycemic index of 64.

There is accumulating evidence that a common diabetic medication called metformin (Glucophage) has an anticancer effect.[8,9] Unlike insulin or other diabetic medications, metformin works by reducing blood insulin levels. Animal studies using mice infected with prostate cancer showed a 50% decrease in cell viability in the animals treated with metformin.[10] This drug is well tolerated and is very familiar to medical practitioners because it has been on the market for decades. If ongoing research confirms these initial observations, metformin may become another effective method for slowing cancer growth.

Thomas's diet reduced insulin so effectively that his body started burning fat as an energy source, resulting in rapid weight loss. Unfortunately, few among us can muster the willpower to follow Thomas's strict regimen of diet and lifestyle. A recent book, *The China Study*, written by Dr. Colin Campbell from Columbia University, suggests that adherence to a straightforward vegan diet, a diet having less than 10% of calories from animal protein, also results in a dramatic reduction in cancer risk. This important book is discussed more fully in chapter 20.

Macrobiotic and vegan diets have many similarities. By avoiding processed foods, macrobiotic diets characteristically have a low glycemic index. Strict macrobiotic diets also include very little animal protein. Amino acids that make up animal protein stimulate insulin release just like glucose does, and animal protein has other growth-stimulating effects.

It causes increased production of insulin-like growth factor, a derivative of growth hormone. Also, as amino acids are essential structural components of new cells, lowering dietary intake creates a "building materials deficiency state," which impedes the creation of new cells.

Strung together like beads on a long chain, amino acids are the basic building blocks of enzymes and structural proteins. To synthesize functional new proteins for cell growth all twenty amino acids must be available in proper amounts. The exact order and how each individual amino acid is located in the chain are specified by DNA via the genetic code. If even one amino acid is absent or out of place, synthesis of the chain ceases and that protein is rendered nonfunctional. To keep this from happening, the replicating cell delays cell division until every last chemical component has been stored up inside the cell ready for use.

Why can't the cancer cells simply make their own amino acids to fulfill their growth needs? Eight of the twenty amino acids are termed "essential" because human cells are unable to synthesize them. The only source of essential amino acids is *from the diet*. Cancer cells are under the same constraints as other human cells. Only by eating animal protein do the cancer cells receive a superabundance of all the essential amino acids, creating a rich "well-fertilized" environment for them to replicate.

In our protein-indoctrinated society my patients usually have the following reaction: "If I eat this way, how will I survive without protein?" The food industry has brainwashed us to believe that eating animal protein is essential for day-to-day survival. Actually, there are plenty of essential amino acids in plants, just not the same overabundance. Our normal cells can meet all their daily requirements from plant protein or by scavenging essential amino acids from the normal turnover of dying cells that have lived out their usefulness and are being replaced. For example, a 150-pound man has more than twenty-five pounds of essential amino acids scattered throughout the normal cells of his body.

Advocates of the macrobiotic diet have their own theories about why the diet works. In the early years, practitioners noticed that a good response to the diet was more likely when body secretions—tears, urine and saliva—became less acidic (they used litmus paper to test the acidity). They concluded that excess acidity in the excreted body fluids meant more acidity inside the body and that acidity was causing cancer to grow. This theory was developed long before the powerful acid/base buffering system of the blood was discovered. We now know that blood pH is immutably fixed at 7.4. Even small changes in pH, a sustained rise above 7.6 or a drop below 7.2, cause death.

Excess acid in the urine or tears does not mean that our blood is more acidic. It just means that the body is dumping acid to maintain a stable internal environment. Unfortunately, to this day, based on observations and conclusions arrived at more than fifty years ago, macrobiotic experts recommend avoiding certain "acidic" foods like tomatoes even though well-designed medical studies indicate that tomatoes are innocuous or even beneficial. This ill-founded fear of acidity has also led to a whole industry that markets worthless products such as low-acid drinking water.

How then can we explain the observations of macrobiotic practitioners who have noted through experience that people with more acidic secretions are less likely to respond to the macrobiotic diet? The answer is fairly simple. Many who claim to be following a rigorous vegan diet either consciously or unconsciously compromise. Surreptitious intake of animal protein (amino acids) is detected in bodily secretions as excess acidity. Acidity does not in itself cause cancer growth; acidity is simply a dietary indicator of something that does—animal protein.

Thomas's commitment to a macrobiotic diet proved remarkably effective. A repeat prostate biopsy in late 2004 revealed less extensive disease than when he was originally diagnosed. His PSA remained low and stable. In late 2007, six years after his initial diagnosis, another biopsy showed that his *Intermediate-Risk* disease was still present but unchanged. In early 2008, he decided to have a radioactive seed implantation. A year later his PSA is declining at the expected rate.

Thomas Mueller's decision to delay radiation and surgery at such a young age may be considered reckless by some members of the medical establishment. But Thomas offers the following rationale: "The pace of advancing medical technology encouraged me to wait as long as possible. I expected less drastic alternatives to surgery and radiation to eventually become available, and so far for me, the seed implant has caused minimal problems. I believe that my diet contributed to keeping my cancer in check all those years."

There are a number of studies confirming that men who overeat and who are overweight display increased incidence and aggressiveness of prostate cancer.[11,12,13,14] However, it now appears that insulin and animal protein are the real culprits. The idea of maintaining low insulin in the blood as the underlying strategy for controlling cancer growth has been poorly understood and has not received the attention it deserves. This failure has resulted in diverse theories and conflicting medical recommendations concerning the role of diet in the treatment of cancer. One thing seems certain: careful attention to the right type of diet is obligatory. Macrobiotic or vegan diets that limit sudden spikes in blood sugar caused by processed foods keep the cancer cells strapped for energy by lowering insulin. These diets also block access to rich sources of essential amino acids, the basic building blocks of replicating cancer cells.

THE PATIENT'S VIEW

The raw science Mark presents here is intriguing and warrants further prospective studies. From the beginning, I had been told that testosterone drove my cancer. Putting the spotlight on insulin activity was an eye-opener. Nevertheless, in Thomas Mueller's case we are witnessing a level of discipline rarely encountered outside a monastery. There are some rare souls who conscientiously adhere to this rigorous lifestyle. An actor friend of mine with prostate cancer is radically committed to diet and exercise as his sole form of cancer therapy; as a result, his body is pure sinew and muscle. His commitment to dietary restraint is remarkable. After ten years of self-denial, his low, stable PSA is to be envied. In my own life, I take inspiration from people like Thomas and my actor friend, and do the best I can.

19.

HEXING: THE MODERN SORCERER'S CURSE

hex n. An evil spell; a curse; used to harm instead of heal. Considered
to be a self-fulfilling prophecy, a prediction of an event due to a strong
belief in the outcome.

—*Free Online Medical Dictionary*

The old adage "Sticks and stones can break my bones but words can never
hurt me" turns out to be dead wrong. Words have tremendous power to
inflict harm. What we say to ourselves, and what is said to us by figures of
authority at critical moments, can produce actual physical consequences.
Expressions like "scared to death," and "worried sick," we now know, are
more than hyperbole. They actually belong to the insidious, primitive behavior known as "hexing."*

It was Andrew Weil, MD, who first brought *medical* hexing to our attention, pointing out that it was a daily occurrence practiced by the entire
medical profession in hospitals, clinics and doctors' offices. Weil called
this behavior "unconscionable," a term defined in *The Concise Oxford
Dictionary* as "not guided or restrained by conscience."

At its most reprehensible, medical hexing becomes a form of "iatro-
genics" (from the Greek *iatros* meaning "physician" and *genic,* meaning
"caused by"), the term used to identify physician- or drug-induced illness,
attributable, at least in part, to negative suggestions by doctors, drug companies or other health care authorities.

To some extent, physicians and pharmaceutical companies are in a bind.
Out-of-control malpractice suits have obliged them to protect themselves

---

* I am indebted to my friend Victor Gurewich, MD, of Harvard Medical School, for
reminding me of an early article on this subject by Harvard physiologist Walter Bradford
Cannon, MA, MD. Entitled "Voodoo Death" and published in *American Anthropologist*
in 1942 (vol. 44: 169–181), the article presents Dr. Cannon's proposed explanation of the
physiological underpinnings of this phenomenon, to which he applied his own graphic
and serviceable term "calamitous imposition."

legally. Before surgery, for instance, patients are required by law to sign an informed consent form that describes everything that could conceivably go wrong as a result of the procedure. And the form you receive from your pharmacist, along with your drug prescription, usually contains an extensive list of warnings about the drug's possible appalling side effects. The problem is that in some people's minds, these warnings become the stuff of self-fulfilling prophecy—the equivalent of a voodoo curse.

FROM VOODOO BONES TO STETHOSCOPES

If a witch doctor leaped out of the jungle, spun around, pointed a bone at you and told you that you were going to die, you'd probably laugh, albeit a trifle nervously. But that's not the case in remote or primitive cultures, where the unfortunate recipient of the curse actually drops dead, presumably of fright. In the current medical environment, however, the traditional voodoo curse appears to have taken on a new life.

In their very practical book, *The Worst Is Over*, Judith Acosta, LCSW, and Judith Simon Prager, PhD, describe how the stress of a medical crisis or emotional trauma, such as a diagnosis of cancer, throws patients into an "altered state" in which they are particularly open to suggestion, good or bad. And because most of us, as children, are taught to believe in the infallibility of doctors, the manner in which a doctor delivers any life-threatening diagnosis actually has the power to influence the course of the disease.

During those critical intake moments, the doctor's words are heard at a very deep level and have a profound impact. If his words are positive, they plant within us positive expectations that we can beat the cancer, that we will be cured. Unfortunately, the reverse is also true. When we are in this altered state, the doctor can literally scare us to death by quoting negative statistics, relating the gruesome side effects of various treatments, or worse, by his use the of dreaded word "terminal."

Although we may joke about voodoo curses, when a modern-day witch doctor wearing a white coat, carrying a stethoscope, and supported by scans and test results, tells you you're going to die, his "curse" may significantly raise the chances that you actually *will* die. It must be said, however, that such a moment provides the perfect opportunity to remember that there is, in surgeon Atul Gawande's words, "an art to being a patient," and practicing that art must include protecting yourself against hexing in any form.

A CASE OF HEXING IN MY OWN CAMP

Reel back in time. It is September 1997, three weeks after Jeanne had undergone a total thyroidectomy. We had been summoned to the office of her endocrinologist at Columbia Presbyterian Hospital in New York City. We were barely seated in his office when, without any effort to prepare us or lessen the blow, the doctor said to Jeanne, "I'm sorry. I have some bad news for you. You fall into the one percent of all thyroidectomy patients who do not properly respond to replacement hormone medication."

In other words, there was no thyroid treatment to keep Jeanne alive. We sat there looking at each other, speechless. So he repeated the ominous words, adding, "If you ever wanted to go to India, get on a plane and go!"

Although Jeanne was numb with shock, she was more angry than frightened. As we left the doctor's office, she turned to me and said, "Well, that's *his* opinion. And he can shove it up his Taj Mahal!"

"So what are you going to do?" I asked her.

Jeanne said, "I'm going to bloody well figure out how to live!"

And she did. But that's another story.

Unfortunately, not everyone possesses Jeanne Blum's survival resources, her medical knowledge and her fighting spirit. And so some people actually do proceed to die on schedule.

HEXING FOR THE UNCONSCIOUS

Words can have an equally powerful impact whether we are physically conscious or not. In fact, when we are unconscious, it appears that we are especially open to suggestion. In his book *Be Careful What You Pray For . . . You Just Might Get It*, Larry Dossey, MD, relates how a patient developed complications after successful abdominal surgery and told a nurse he felt he was going to die. A psychiatrist was called in, and while hypnotized, the patient recalled that when he was under the anesthetic he heard someone say, "This is the worst case I've ever seen." He believed what he had heard and coming out of the surgery, he immediately began to decline. As it turned out, a fourth-year medical student had indeed spoken those words. But he had seen only one other case and had meant his remark as a joke. Once the med student had explained his comment to the patient, the man completely recovered.

We've all heard stories of people in comas who heard everything that was said around them but couldn't respond. A considerable amount has been written about unconscious patients actually taking in operating room chatter, some of it sick humor, à la M*A*S*H. Because their normal defense mechanisms are not functioning, they are unusually vulnerable to promiscuous medical hexing.

There can, however, be a positive side to this operating room "eavesdropping." For years, Dr. Bernie Siegel has been talking reassuringly to anesthetized patients in order to ward off and prevent complications in the operating room. In his first book, *Love, Medicine & Miracles*, he writes about reversing cardiac irregularities and slowing the pulse rate of patients during surgery by giving them calming instructions. My favorite Siegel moment—a rather dramatic "Jesus moment"—took place after the heart of an obese young male patient named Harry had stopped beating and he had not responded to resuscitation efforts. The anesthesiologist had already given up and was leaving the OR when, in a loud voice, Siegel said, "Harry, it's *not* your time. Come on back!" As if on cue, the cardiogram began to show electrical activity, and the young man did, indeed, return.

MEET THE PLACEBO'S EVIL TWIN

"If we look ahead far enough, we can see that placebos may be the best medicine of all." So wrote Deepak Chopra, in his book *Creating Health*.

Everyone has heard of the placebo effect, the beneficial results that a sugar pill or some sham medical procedure can produce if the patient is told by his doctor that it will bring relief or healing. However, the placebo (Latin for "I will please") has a lesser-known evil twin, the *nocebo* (Latin for "I will harm"), which produces just the opposite results and causes the patient to suffer damaging side effects. Either because of the negative words of his doctor, or because he is frightened by dire warnings of a drug's potential side effects, the patient believes that something bad is going to happen, and all too often it does. Thus, according to Dr. Siegel, it is the "expectations aroused" in the patient that ultimately determine the outcome.

It is hard for most people living in the twenty-first century to imagine, let alone believe, that our beliefs can kill us. Or heal us. It's even harder to convince some doctors that a patient's problems may be more than just physical. In his book *Placebo-Effect Healing: The Power and Biology of Belief,* Dr. Herbert Benson, MD, marvels at how the medical community undervalues the significance of the placebo effect, which he describes as "the ability of a person to affect his or her physiological well-being with just a thought."

As to why we do not have better data concerning the nocebo effect, as one doctor put it, "It is difficult to obtain either ethical approval or willing volunteers for studies designed to make people feel worse."

Nor are these simply psychological phenomena. It is now known from PET scans (scans that can detect changes in the body at the cellular level) that both placebos and nocebos produce measurable consequences that are recorded in brain activity. But bottom line, although it is our thoughts and our beliefs that create the cascade of chemicals that can either harm or heal us, it is often the doctor who starts the process. And when the doctor arouses negative expectations, that qualifies as medical hexing.

I read recently about a man who was diagnosed with end-stage liver cancer. His doctor gave him just months to live, and he duly died in the allotted time frame. Then an autopsy revealed that the doctor had gotten it wrong: the man's tumor was extremely small, and there was no sign of metastasis. Apparently the patient had not died from cancer, but from *believing* he was dying of cancer.

Welcome to witch doctor country!

SELF-HEXING

When you are diagnosed with any type of cancer it's natural to ask, "Why did this happen to me?" And if you don't ask it consciously, the question is probably there, lurking somewhere beneath the surface, along with other questions like, "Could I have prevented it?" or "Did I do something to bring it on myself?" There are no easy answers. However, sometimes the answers we give ourselves are based on guilt, not reality. The more I've learned about this disease the more I realize that cancer is as much a psychological and spiritual challenge as a physical one.

To some extent we are all responsible for our own health, but there are people who cross the line from responsibility to guilt and self-blame. No evidence exists to indicate that prostate cancer is some sort of involuntary atonement for past behavior. Yet on several occasions when I was inter-viewing for this book, I heard confessions of guilt from men who secretly believed that their prostate cancer was punishment for sexual misconduct, for having been "bad boys." I regard this as a form of self-hexing.

Invariably these were intelligent, rational men who occupied respon-sible positions in the world. And yet, although they rarely discussed it, these men were convinced that their promiscuity was a factor in getting prostate cancer. Or as one man put it, "catching the cancer," as if it were some kind of venereal disease. Irrational? Maybe. But in keeping with the ancient notions in ethics and law as far back as Deuteronomy—the "eye for an eye" formula, the just measure of "let the punishment fit the crime."

My first encounter with someone who was practicing self-hexing came in 2006 at a men's retreat in Sarasota Springs, California. I was sitting under the stars in a hot tub with a fifty-four-year-old veterinary surgeon, Jack Menzies, when we got onto the subject of prostates. Jack sounded depressed. It turned out that nine months earlier he'd had surgery for pros-tate cancer and was struggling with ongoing urinary and impotence prob-lems. It struck me that at fifty-four, that was enough to depress anyone. But Jack had different concerns.

"I'll be perfectly straight with you," he said. "I went through a long period when I was really promiscuous, I mean *years*. I've had three wives, and I cheated on all of them." He paused, turned on the hot tub jets, then said, "I guess I got what I deserved!"

On rare occasions self-hexing can pave the way to redemption. Several years ago, at a Prostate Cancer Research Institute Conference, I met a Catholic priest, Father Dave, who, although he was living with metasta-sized prostate cancer, seemed to me to be totally at peace with himself.

"Before entering the priesthood I was a committed sex addict," Father Dave told me. "Nowadays, I think of the ancient curse and prediction from Scripture, Matthew 26:52, our Lord's words to Peter: 'All those who have taken up the sword shall perish by the sword.' What if, for 'sword' you read 'penis'? Somehow it made sense to me that my prostate cancer was my fault. No, better say, my penance. Even though I had confessed my sins and received absolution, and even though I knew God had forgiven me, in my own eyes, my own secret heart, I remained weighed down with guilt, and the cancer was my way of atoning, of redeeming myself through suffering so that *I* could forgive myself. God's forgiveness wasn't enough."

He smiled at me. "Sounds like another sin altogether, doesn't it? Aren't we funny creatures?"

At last report, Father Dave was still saying Mass and counseling men newly diagnosed with prostate cancer.

Finally, there is the painful, yet totally irrational self-hexing by the innocent. While I was writing this chapter, I mentioned it to an Irish friend who prefers to remain anonymous because he is still dealing with what happened. He told me he had always wondered whether being assaulted at the age of twelve by his French teacher, Mr. Nester, on a field trip to France, might explain why he developed prostate cancer.

"He tried to jerk me off at a chateau in the South of France," my friend told me. "The poor bastard wanted to make me his loveboy."

"So what did you do?"

"What did I do? I fled. I hitchhiked back to Dublin. And do you know, somehow I felt that what happened was *my* fault. I never mentioned that experience out loud, not once. Not to my father, not to my mother, not to my wife, not to my analyst. For more than forty years, not a word! Then a couple of years ago, when I already had prostate cancer, I was getting a treatment from an acupuncturist, and suddenly it became imperative that I speak it out loud. What a relief! And what I ask myself now is, had I been able to speak about it years ago, might my doing so have averted the cancer?"

Nor is self-hexing exclusive to men. According to psychologist Carolyn Conger, women experience the same agonies of guilt and self-blame.

"I've listened to a number of women confess that they felt they deserved their cancers," Carolyn told me. "Most touching was a client who said, 'I let too many strangers into my body. Now, with the hysterectomy, I feel I've lost my womanhood.' Of course this is not logical. Femininity is not localized in the womb any more than masculinity is localized in the prostate."

And yet how many men believe that the prostate gland is *all* about masculinity, especially when surgery, radiation or chemical castration (aka hormone therapy) threatens their ability to perform? As for me, I no longer regard my ability to get erections as the hallmark of my masculinity. When all is said and done, I know that living all these years with prostate cancer has strengthened my sense of myself as a man. I don't remember giving any thought to *why* I got prostate cancer. Had I considered it at all, I would probably have assumed that the Angel of Death had delivered the cancer to the wrong door. And although I have logged many miles as a bad boy, either through good luck or denial, it never occurred to me to connect the cancer to my less than exemplary sexual history. As a result, I reckon I have been spared the feelings of guilt and self-blame that negatively impact the immune system—our most powerful ally in the cancer wars.

REFRAMING: AN ANTIDOTE TO SELF-HEXING

The degree to which I may have participated in getting prostate cancer is a question I can't answer. There are so many potential contributing factors that it's impossible to nail any one culprit. Moreover, that's not what's important, other than as a recognition that I can also participate in my own healing. What I know for sure is that for me, cancer has been a serious wake-up call.

I can see now that the way I was living for so many years made me a likely candidate for some life-threatening disease. Simply put, I did not take good care of my health. Neither was I aware of the intangible factors that can make so much difference. I spent a lot of time regretting the past, fearing the future and not appreciating the present. It seems I needed a shock to jolt me awake, to bring me to my senses. There's an old story about the professor of animal husbandry who enters his classroom one morning leading a mule by a rope and carrying a baseball bat. "Today, class," he says, "we will consider the care and handling of the mule," with which, he drops the rope, winds up with his bat, and delivers a crashing blow to the animal's head. The mule shudders violently, its legs go stiff, its eyes bug out. The professor turns to his class and says, "First, you have to get the mule's attention." Prostate cancer was my baseball bat.

However, once I was over the initial shock, instead of regarding the cancer as a threat to my life, I was able to see it as a heads up, an urgent message from my body signaling that I needed to review and reshape my life on all levels—physical, emotional and spiritual. "Reframing" the cancer, finding a positive way of responding to it as a catalyst for change, lessened my fear by shifting my focus to what I could do to begin healing myself. And as I learned more about our ability to tilt the scales toward either healing or illness with our thoughts and beliefs, I became increasingly aware that men who blamed themselves for getting cancer were hurting their chances of recovery.

THE SELF-HEXER'S COCKTAIL

By the dim light of ecclesiastical self-blame and guilt (Father Dave's "perish by the sword" homily), I offer the following "metaphorical" Italian cocktail (*aperitivo metaforico*). The "cocktail" recipe I am including for your delectation was allegedly found in the discarded codpiece of a certain Prince of the Church after his untimely demise (from prostate cancer, it is believed) in the arms of his mistress, the Countess Benedetta Borgia (1604–1653).

Although I googled her, I could find no Countess, Borgia or otherwise, bearing that name or living in that period. I almost chucked the cocktail out as fraudulent. But I held back. And finally I think I see purpose in this metaphorical concoction. The somewhat pedestrian translation from the Italian is my own, as is the more contemporary name for the draught.

THE SELF-HEXER'S COCKTAIL
Combine the following ingredients:

1 finger (un ditto) *of abject fear*
1 finger of self-doubt
3 tablespoons (cucchiae) *of resentful anger*
56 grams of profound regret
1 finger or 2 each (cada uno) *of jealousy and self-pity*
4 generous parts (portzioni generosi) *unrelieved guilt*
Add despair and anxiety to taste

Mix ingredients while brooding and moaning over your distressing situation (tears of despair are optional for flavor) and drink when feeling especially vulnerable.

Well, there you have it, my rave about hexing. To all the "bad boys" who are sabotaging their recovery by wallowing in guilt and indulging in self-blame, I would say: Don't waste a moment! Now is the time to consider the toxic effects of self-hexing and forgive yourselves. Forgiveness, along with love and gratitude, ranks right at the top on every list of essential requirements for mind–body healing.

Ultimately, there is no logic to support the belief that *any* disease is self-punishing atonement for past "sins," let alone that it is retribution from on high. Ironically, it may well be as Italian playwright Luigi Pirandello put it: *Cosi e si vi pare*, "Right you are if you think you are."

All too often what you believe is what you attract.

DOCTOR'S VIEW

Unfortunately what Ralph describes is all too common. Time and again I have been dismayed to hear how my patients were told by their doctors that they only had a specified amount of time to live, the danger, of course, being the influence this could have on the real prognosis. Patients need to guard against and reject such Olympian pronouncements. No one knows the future with absolute precision. Patients and health care providers alike forget that the only resources doctors have for giving a prognosis—for predicting the future—are medical studies. The problem is that medical studies report averages for groups of patients. At best, they provide only a rough sense of various, possible future outcomes. They cannot be relied upon to accurately predict the future for a specific individual. Ever.

20.

DIET AND SUPPLEMENTS: AN OVERVIEW

You Are What You Eat

—VICTOR LINDLAHR

Each man's prostate cancer grows at a genetically predetermined rate. However, the growth rate can also be influenced by external factors. The same is true of all living things. Crops grow faster when we provide plenty of fertilizer and water. Children in our Western culture tend to grow bigger and taller due to our high-protein diet. Fortunately, even with unhealthy diets, prostate cancer tends to grow slowly.

For many men, a diagnosis of prostate cancer is a wake-up call to make important lifestyle and dietary changes. Basically there are two goals. First, slow the rate of prostate cancer growth and thus delay treatment as long as possible. Second, use the diagnosis as motivation for improving overall basic health practices. One of my patients, Gary Driggs, has written a pamphlet titled, "How Prostate Cancer Can Extend Your Life." His message is the same as that conveyed by the famous medical statistician Dr. Michael Kattan, who wrote in the *Journal of Urology* in January 2006, "Age, fitness, and body weight have a far bigger effect on survival than PSA, Gleason score, or any type of treatment. The diagnosis of prostate cancer should be taken as a helpful wake-up call encouraging men to improve their diet and start exercising."

Once diagnosed with prostate cancer men frequently start taking an avid interest in supplements. The supplement and vitamin industry is huge. Many companies hawk substances claiming that they stimulate the immune system. Studies in Petri dishes or in animals are often used to support their claims. But these studies are misleading or outright deceptive because controlling cancer in a Petri dish or in a rat does not mean that the same substance will control cancer in people. I have seen rats cured of cancer over and over. Only rarely do these "huge breakthroughs" translate into useful treatments for people. If we want to determine which studies should be believed and which should be ignored, a good beginning place is to disregard the animal and laboratory studies altogether. Results from these "studies" are merely exploratory, never conclusive.

Unfortunately, because of the many outlandish claims, some patients give up on science altogether. Disillusioned, they conclude that nothing can be known with certainty. This is an extreme position and ignores the fact that *human* studies give important insights into what promotes health and what inhibits prostate cancer. Although human studies are not perfect, when two separate and completely independent research groups come to the same conclusion, their findings can probably be trusted.

Before I review what we know and don't know about diet and supplements, let's address a deceptive and misleading myth used repeatedly as a marketing scheme—the idea that the medical industry is suppressing some marvelous cure because it competes with other more expensive medicines that the pharmaceutical industry is trying to foist on you. These conspiracy theories are ridiculous when you consider that we live in a free world. There are millions of men living with prostate cancer who are on the lookout for a cure. It is impossible to hide effective treatment from so many motivated people. Even so, I see people fall for this foolish ploy all the time.

Let me give you an example of how quickly word spreads when an effective product does come along. PC-SPES, a formula of Chinese herbs invented by a scientist named Sophie Chen, came on the market as a nonprescription over-the-counter supplement in the mid-1990s (Ralph described his experience with PC-SPES in chapter 3). I still remember the day my office got an excited call from someone in Florida. "My PSA has dropped from 200 down to 30. I've been taking a pill called PC-SPES." Only a few days later we received a second call, this time from a man in New York, "My PSA has dropped from 25 down to 4. I think it's from an herb called PC-SPES."

We contacted the manufacturer of PC-SPES and offered to study the substance in our patients. The company obliged, providing us with free pills for testing purposes. After evaluating it in about a dozen men we confirmed that it was indeed effective and that it appeared to work by lowering testosterone via an estrogenic effect. We also discovered that like most effective anticancer agents there were side effects. PC-SPES, similar to estrogen, could induce breast enlargement and cause blood clots. Subsequently Dr. Eric Small at the University of California at San Francisco performed a more elaborate randomized study, which indicated that PC-SPES was better than estrogen in a head-to-head trial.

Unfortunately, several years later, the company that made PC-SPES was sued for purportedly adulterating the product with prescription pharmaceuticals. The company took the product off the maket and the lawsuits are ongoing to this day. However, the point is this: *when an effective treatment comes along, word spreads fast.*

DIET

How diet affects cancer growth was discussed in chapter 18. It amazes me how often this critically important topic is underemphasized. Yet the statistics are overwhelming. Mortality rates from prostate cancer are eighteen times lower in the Far East than in the United States.[1] Genetic differences cannot explain these statistics because when Asians move to the United States and start eating our Western diet, mortality rates start rising. Our National Cancer Institute has spent millions of dollars researching diet in China. China was selected for the research because most people born there grow up, live and die in the same place. They rarely move around and their dietary habits remain stable throughout their lives. This means that researchers can study disease patterns in different parts of the country and compare the frequency of certain illnesses in each area with the prevalent type of diet. A beautiful summary of these extensive studies has been published in a book called *The China Study*, by Colin Campbell. The most important finding of these studies was that the more animal protein you eat, the higher your risk of dying of cancer.

Even before I learned about Dr. Campbell's book, my own experience with patients had taught me the importance of diet. On several occasions men with rising PSA levels from relapsed cancer proposed treating their cancer with diet alone. I couldn't help but sit up and take notice when, usually within a couple of months, their steadily rising PSA levels would suddenly stabilize. Typically these men were following a macrobiotic approach. Dr. Campbell's research is not the only data pointing to the importance of diet. A plethora of studies performed here in the United States conclude that being overweight and overeating lead to an increased incidence or an increased aggressiveness of prostate cancer.[2,3] It appears that the epidemic levels of cancer in the United States are primarily a result of our poor eating habits.

SPECIFIC FOODS

One frequently studied candidate is soy. After all, it's a major component of the Asian diet and the fact that people living in Asia have less cancer is indisputable. The active ingredients in soy are genistein and daidzein, which act to inhibit cell growth and new blood vessel formation. Various epidemiologic studies show a reduced incidence of prostate cancer with increased soy intake.[4,5,6] However, enthusiasm for loading up on soy has slowed down quickly since a study was published relating excess soy to Alzheimer's.[7]

Another food that has received much attention is pomegranate juice. A preliminary trial in fifty men with increasing PSA levels showed a significant slowing in the rate of PSA rise after starting on a regime of pomegranate juice. Based on these promising early results, a multi-center trial at several famous institutions around the country is ongoing and a final and definitive answer should be available about the time this book is published. The same company that is sponsoring the trial, the manufacturer of POM Wonderful, has created a pomegranate pill, which may be a healthier alternative for daily use as it contains much less sugar.

Though certain foods may turn out to be helpful, other foods are clearly deleterious. As previously discussed, animal protein, particularly in the form of red meat, has been associated with an increasing incidence of prostate cancer.[8] Red meat contains more than 50% fat and high-fat diets increase the level of insulin-like growth factor,[9] which in turn increases the risk of prostate cancer.[10,11] Of all the different types of animal protein, fish seems to be the safest. In fact, two studies have been published showing a protective effect from eating fish.[12,13] This benefit is thought to originate from the high content of marine omega-3 fatty acids, which can also be obtained through supplements.

The most important principle I have learned about what makes a diet effective is this: "it's not what you eat, *it's what you abstain from eating.*"

MILK

Milk is the ideal growth food for infants but not for adults. It is high in calcium but also high in fat and has been associated with a higher incidence of prostate cancer progression.[14,15] Milk also stimulates increased production of insulin-like growth factor,[16] which is associated with more aggressive cancer behavior. Another component of milk that may be of concern is phytanic acid, a complex fatty acid that is also present in red meat. Prostate cancer cells overproduce an enzyme called AMACR, which metabolizes phytanic acid, providing needed energy for growth.[17] Phytanic acid metabolism also releases hydrogen peroxide, a toxic byproduct that can cause oxidative damage leading to cell mutations (see below). As if that weren't enough, milk also contains casein, the ultimate animal protein. Casein includes every essential amino acid in perfect proportion for the encouragement of rapid cancer growth.

Cancer replication slows when the raw materials for building new cells are unavailable. While the normal cells in our adult bodies can scavenge essential amino acids from other dying cells, cancer cells need an abundant oversupply to proliferate. Animal proteins—meats, milk, cheese and eggs—fuel the pace of cancer cell growth.

ANTIOXIDANTS

Prostate cancer starts with DNA mutations, often caused by oxygen free radicals, a byproduct of inflammation. We know that oxygen free radicals are important because the main enzyme that protects our cells from them—glutathione transferase—is almost invariably inactivated in cancer cells. Apparently, it is very difficult for prostate cancer to arise unless this protective enzyme has been inactivated.

The theory that DNA mutations are caused by oxygen free radicals is also supported by human studies showing a reduced incidence of prostate cancer in men eating diets rich in antioxidants. For example, eating tomato sauce, which is high in lycopene, the most common antioxidant found in the prostate, reduces the risk of developing advanced prostate cancer by as much as 35%.[18] Higher serum lycopene levels in the blood have been associated with up to an 80% reduction in the risk of being diagnosed with prostate cancer. A meta-analysis—a compilation of multiple studies measuring the amount of tomatoes in the diet, particularly cooked tomatoes—showed a 20% reduction in prostate cancer risk with increased consumption.[19]

Along with lycopene, selenium displays strong antioxidant properties. An essential trace element, selenium comes from both plant and animal sources. Brazil nuts are noted for their unusually high selenium content (approximately 500 mcg per ounce) as are clams, turkey and mushrooms. Higher levels of selenium in the blood are associated with a 50% reduction in the incidence of prostate cancer.[20]

Enthusiasm for the benefits of selenium and lycopene may need to be tempered somewhat considering a recent study published in the *Journal of the National Cancer Institute* that showed no change in the frequency of diagnosing prostate cancer within the first five years after starting supplementation.[21] However, in my opinion the main flaw of the study was that it looked at a mere five-year time period, which is not reflective of the twenty-to-forty-year period that men harbor prostate cancer before diagnosis. Also, despite evaluating over thirty thousand men, only two, whether they were on these supplements or not, actually died of prostate cancer.

Vitamin E, a strong antioxidant, is often touted for its protective effects against prostate cancer. Several studies have shown up to a 40% reduction in prostate cancer risk with the use of vitamin E. One study in particular showed benefit using a relatively small daily dose of only 50 IU.[22] However, enthusiasm for using vitamin E is waning. A compilation of multiple vitamin E studies showed that excessive vitamin E caused more harm than good. There was an *increase* in mortality with the use of 400 IU daily compared to the people who were not taking it.[23] Another study indicates that vitamin E should be avoided by individuals taking cholesterol pills. This study, published in the *New England Journal of Medicine,* showed that vitamin E negated the cholesterol-lowering effect of these pharmaceuticals.[24]

Before leaving the antioxidant topic, I want to mention one last food group, the cruciferous vegetables (such as broccoli, cauliflower, Brussels sprouts and cabbage), which have also been associated with a 50% reduction in prostate cancer risk.[25] A substance called sulforaphane appears to be the most active ingredient in these vegetables. Sulforaphane itself is not a direct antioxidant. Rather, sulforaphane works by stimulating the cells to manufacture more of the protective antioxidant enzyme glutathione transferase, which is usually suppressed or inactivated in cancer cells.

VITAMIN D

A number of convincing lines of evidence show that vitamin D inhibits prostate cancer growth. Vitamin D in the blood increases with sun exposure, and studies show that mortality rates from prostate cancer decrease as exposure to ultraviolet light increases. However, melanin in the skin reduces the synthesis of vitamin D, which may partially explain why African Americans have a higher incidence and higher mortality from prostate cancer than Caucasians. In studies using pharmacologic doses of synthetic vitamin D in men with relapsed prostate cancer, PSA levels stabilized and even declined in some men.[26] Despite its proven benefits, vitamin D deficiency is common in the general population, perhaps because we limit sun exposure due to concerns about skin cancer. As a result, the minimum dose should probably exceed 1000 IU daily.[27] A more effective method is to check the levels of vitamin D in the blood and increase the dose until high-normal blood levels are achieved.

CALCIUM

High doses of calcium, in amounts exceeding 2000 mg daily, have been associated in multiple studies with an elevated risk of prostate cancer.[14,28] In one study, a 400% increase in calcium intake was associated with an increased incidence of metastatic disease,[29] whereas doses of 1000 mg a day or less have *not* been linked to increased risk. It's difficult to know if the adverse effects of high-dose calcium result from stimulating cancer growth directly or if it's a secondary effect of excess calcium lowering vitamin D, which calcium is known to do when it is in excess.

MULTIVITAMINS AND MINERALS

The results of a well-designed study of high doses of multivitamins published in the *Journal of the National Cancer Institute* indicated a higher risk of prostate cancer mortality with excess intake of multivitamins.[30] Similar problems have been reported with zinc, iron and copper supplementation.[31] I advise cancer patients to avoid multivitamin and multimineral preparations, as in some cases they may accelerate cancer growth.

FINAL THOUGHTS

The fact that taking a pill is so much easier than making major dietary or lifestyle changes easily explains the existence of the multibillion-dollar supplement industry. Rather than addressing the hard question of how to change our diet and lower our intake of animal protein, we swallow a pill. Dietary research of the quality and scope reported in *The China Study,* in which people's eating patterns over a lifetime were evaluated, is unlikely to be replicated. Research into the effects of a pill or supplement is much easier and cheaper to perform. Therefore, expect the media to continue barraging us with reports of new studies of some individual food, vitamin or supplement that purportedly has special anticancer effects. The current fad as I write, is asparagus. Enjoy asparagus but don't be fooled by the hype. Common sense dictates that the diet we choose, a diet low in calories and animal protein, is vastly more important for controlling cancer than the impact of any specific pill or supplement.

Table 6. Recommended Supplements*

Calcium 500 mg with dinner
Fish oil 1000 mg twice a day
Vitamin D 2000 IU daily
Lycopene 10 mg daily
To be avoided: multivitamins, iron, copper and zinc

* A list is at best a general guideline because individual needs vary.

THE PATIENT'S VIEW

Nowadays, threatened with overwhelming floods of information on just about everything, we benefit hugely from data management and reduction by someone who knows the material, especially sensible advice on what supplements to take, what to eat and, more to the point, what not to eat. In the early years of my prostate cancer, I took PC-SPES and, like thousands of others, was cut adrift when it was taken off the market. I rely on the supplements Mark suggests but I also add my own choices (Resveratrol, Lipoic Acid, DMAE, various jungle roots and barks). I take calcium to make sure my bones are getting some daily supply. And there's this: getting help with choices is a major contribution to stress reduction, for which your immune system will reward you.

21.

ROMANCING THE IMMUNE SYSTEM

Every cell in your body is eavesdropping on your thoughts.

—DEEPAK CHOPRA, MD

The immune system is a wonder. It is multiplex, intricate, and altogether fascinating. However, since I never studied even the basics of any scientific discipline, this briefing will be The Immune System for Dummies.

As I understand it, the immune system is a bodywide network of cells, tissues and organs that has evolved to defend us against foreign invaders. The body's equivalent of the Department of Homeland Security, its primary task is to provide constant surveillance and, when necessary, rally the troops to seek out "terrorists"—defective or cancerous cells—and destroy them.

A healthy immune system will respond to a signal ("flotilla of rogue cancer cells approaching the islets of Langerhans!"*) and will perform its defensive function by immediately going into attack mode ("Launching T cells! . . . Launching natural killer cells!"). However, when immune surveillance breaks down as a result of environmental pollutants, toxins, poor diet, lack of exercise and an array of emotional suppressors, the immune system can no longer do its job. This is when tumors develop. And the irony is the degree to which, all too often, we ourselves are the saboteurs.

When I finally accepted the fact that I had prostate cancer, my ignorance about the immune system was monumental. Mostly I took it for granted. Then, quite recently, I decided to find out what makes my immune system tick; in particular, what disrupts its ability to function efficiently as

---

* Discovered in 1869 by German anatomist pathologist Peter Langerhans, the islets of Langerhans constitute approximately 1 to 2% of the mass of the pancreas. There are about one million islets in a healthy adult human pancreas.

my champion, and how I could support it beyond doing a better job with diet and exercise. That was when I realized that my brain is constantly sending my immune system chemical messages which, for better or worse, influence its ability to function effectively. I began to think of this process as *Emotional-Chemical Text Messaging* (ECTM).

A BRIEF HISTORY OF EMOTIONAL-CHEMICAL TEXT MESSAGING

There is now an immense amount of research documenting the ways mind and body, brain and immune system communicate. In 1964, George Solomon published a landmark article entitled "Emotions, Immunity and Disease: A Speculative Theoretical Integration." Solomon started with a single hypothesis — that "stress can be immunosuppressive." Ten years later, Solomon's findings were no longer regarded as speculative. In 1975 psychiatrist Robert Adler and immunologist Nicholas Cohen coined the nine-syllable tongue-twister of a term, *psychoneuroimmunology*,* a portmanteau word (in effect a "suitcase") into which are packed the essentials for the study of the interaction between psychological processes, the nervous system and the immune system.

In 1981, Adler and Cohen, together with neurobiologist David Felton, wrote a groundbreaking two-volume work entitled *Psychoneuroimmunology* (4th edition, 2006), setting out the premise that the brain and immune system represent a single integrated system of defense.

Pioneering research by neuropharmacologist Candace Pert revealed that the mind and body are one interconnected information system. Start with the idea that body and mind are what Bernie Siegel calls "different expressions of the same information" — information that is carried by messenger molecules known as peptides and neuropeptides from the mind and brain to the body, and then back again, in a continuous feedback loop. As Siegel explains in his admirable book, *Peace, Love & Healing*, peptides "make possible the movement from perception or thought or

---

* Psychoneuroimmunology (PNI) is the study of the interaction between psychological processes and the nervous and immune systems of the human body. PNI takes an interdisciplinary approach, incorporating psychology, neuroscience, immunology, physiology, pharmacology, molecular biology, psychiatry, behavioral medicine, infectious diseases, endocrinology and rheumatology.

feeling in the mind, to messages transmitted by the brain, to hormonal secretions and on down to cellular action in the body" and then back again
in a never-ending feedback loop.

The primary site where body and mind meet through the action of the
peptides is in the limbic/hypothalamic area of the brain where peptide
receptor "hot spots" are located. But there is another hot spot in the linings
of the gut and stomach. So when people say they had a "gut reaction," it
appears to be a physiological truth.

Siegel summed up the whole amazing process in three words when he
famously said, "Feelings are chemical."

YOU CAN DECIDE WHICH EMOTIONAL-CHEMICAL
TEXT MESSAGES TO SEND

Because peptide messenger molecules transmit Emotional-Chemical Text
Messages between brain and body, we can either send messages that evoke
a positive biochemical response in the immune system, or we can send
messages that suppress immune function. As my friend Harvey put it, "For
a time my negative thoughts were interfering with my medication."

Harvey is convinced that, at a critical moment in his cancer treatment,
he turned things around by sending his immune system a positive healing message. When his PSA almost doubled in under three weeks, he was
terrified, depressed, ready to give up.

"I was lying awake in the middle of the night," Harvey told me, "and I
was thinking I'd quit right now, just toss in the sponge, if it weren't for the
children. At that moment, my six-year-old, Jasper, came and crawled into
bed with me. And as he snuggled up I suddenly knew with total clarity: *By
God, I'm going to live! I'm going to get well for the children!* And I swear to
you, Ralph, that thought turned everything around. A week later, my PSA
had fallen by 50%!"

A whole slew of negative emotions—fear, anger, resentment, jealousy,
regret and the like—act to suppress the immune system. But the most
potent immune suppressor is *prolonged emotional stress*—unrelieved grief,
persistent feelings of fear, anxiety and hopelessness that lead to depression.
All of these conditions, in varying degrees, transmit negative Emotional-
Chemical Text Messages to the immune system which, because it possesses no analytical filter, acts on what it is, in effect, "told" by the brain.

Although body cells possess intelligence, their only "knowledge" is the information they receive, which means that the "reality" of our fears or anxieties is neither challenged nor verified. The cells don't check back and ask the brain, "Are you *sure* you want to accept as *truth* that you only have six months to live?" When a threat is recognized, all systems go into the fight-or-flight mode that our ancestors relied upon. However, Nature never intended this "On your mark! Get set! Go!" response to last more than a moment or two. So when the brain sends a threat message for which there is no swift resolution, the fight-or-flight response stays stuck on "Get set!" As a result, the immune system is locked into protection mode and is no longer capable of performing the remedial function that is our most powerful defense against cancer.

Mind you, this is not about denying or suppressing so-called negative emotions. It doesn't mean never expressing anger, never feeling fearful or sad. Quite the opposite. It's when we hold onto anger or grief or fear, or just plain give up, that toxic stress floods the body with adrenaline and cortisone derivatives that act to inhibit immune function. That's the bad news.

The good news is that once we understand how Emotional-Chemical Text Messaging works, we can choose to romance the immune system by sending it messages of hope and peace and, above all, messages of gratitude for the incredible job it does keeping us alive and healthy. And we further do our part by staying, to the utmost of our ability, in the present moment; by overindulging in laughter (even smiles count), by practicing forgiveness and by loving unconditionally.

PARADISE LOST

Until recently, my own process has been primarily one of luck and trust in my instincts. First, I was blessed with the tortoise of cancers rather than the hare. And second, I had no idea at the time that those peaceful nine years I spent on Maui, enjoying my life and not worrying, had supported and even strengthened my immune system and, I am convinced, helped to keep the cancer on hold.

Only then, as the saying goes, we fell on hard times. Jeanne had her own health challenges—diabetes, chronic heart disease, recurring lymphoblastic leukemia, thyroid surgery and a body that rejected thyroid replacement medication—all the poison fruit of having been overradiated as an infant in Bermuda. She might as well have been born in Chernobyl. As she put it, with her wry Brit sense of humor, "Blum and I are just your typical American two-cancer family!"

At the same time, finding ourselves saddled with serious financial problems, Jeanne and I were forced to sell our old plantation house in Haiku and give up the life we loved on Maui. I remember the sadness I felt going out for the last time in an outrigger canoe and shooting a mental movie to replay in the future: the power of the canoe surging over the still surface of the Wailuku bay, sunlight glinting from the sheen of water spilling off our blades as they dipped and rose, dipped and rose, everyone pulling in unison. And afterward, when we dragged the canoe ashore and I made a gift of my paddle to my young Hawaiian friend, Kalani Kalaohe, who had always had to borrow one from the rowing club, I felt a wave of sadness: passing on my paddle marked the end of an era.

That last paddle in the outrigger canoe on Wailuku Bay was when I began to grieve for the passing of an idyllic way of life. Yet even before we made the decision to abandon upcountry Maui and move back to the mainland, Jeanne and I were not doing well; our relationship was going through a rocky patch, and I was chronically stressed and depressed, wondering if I'd been a fool, refusing to commit to treatment that might have resulted in a cure.

All these conditions, I now realize, were red alerts, stressors that acted to inhibit my immune system. And sure enough, that was when my PSA began to climb and the tumor began to grow.

PHYSICAL ENVIRONMENT: DIET AND EXERCISE

Everyone I have talked with who has done really well in the cancer wars has made diet and exercise a key part of their recovery program. So although my own record in these areas barely deserves passing marks, I would be remiss if I didn't at least mention in this chapter the key role good nutrition and staying physically active play in supporting healthy immune function.

The problem for me has been that, like a lot of guys who grew up on steak and fries, I'm not big on raw foods, low carbs or an excess of leafy greens. The idea of a formal macrobiotic diet was foreign to me—and Lord knows, Jeanne tried, but Hawaiian barbecued pork ribs had me sneaking up the road. And if I drank a glass of pure water every waking hour I'd never get more than sprinting distance from the john.

However, there's always hope. In chapter 20, Mark provides sound advice on diet and supplements for men with prostate cancer. Personally, I would recommend Patrick Quillin's *Beating Cancer with Nutrition*. Given his focus on slowing and even reversing cancer growth, he has helped thousands of cancer patients with his excellent nutrition advice. What's more, his book is most helpful in that it provides an extensive list of doctors across this country and around the world who incorporate nutrition into their medical practice.

Given my aversion to all forms of exercise, I wasn't pleased to learn that exercise stimulates the immune system and helps us cope better with stress. On the bright side, you don't have to run marathons or knock yourself out for two hours at the gym every day. When exercise is a chore, it defeats its purpose and becomes one more form of stress. However, according to Dr. Quillin, only 14% of *active* Americans will get cancer. So I am now a regular—well, semiregular—at my local YMCA, which happens to be just two blocks from our door. I get myself there by applying what my friend Carl Bresk, who teaches at the Y, calls "the ten minute rule." I wake up, think about exercising—and turn over and sleep another half hour. But then I hear Carl's voice in my head: "Just *get* yourself to the Y. Make a deal with yourself that you'll stay ten minutes—in the weight room, on the treadmill, in the pool. Only ten minutes!" Some days I make it, some days I don't. But all those ten minutes are slowly adding up.

When I decided to improve my diet and get myself to the Y, Jeanne's comment was, "Think of it as sending your immune system flowers and chocolates—and an occasional ticket to a Lakers game!"

"LIFESTYLE THERAPY"

No matter how dire your prognosis, there is always strong reason for hope *provided* you take an active part in your recovery process. Remember the old rule of the desert: "Trust in God, but tie your camel to a tree." Well, the same applies with a cancer diagnosis. First, find a medical team you trust. Then *your* task is to do everything in your power to contribute to your complete recovery. And that means entering into what longtime cancer survivor and activist Greg Anderson calls "lifestyle therapy."

Before his cancer, Anderson was vice-president and executive director of the Robert Schuller Institute at the Crystal Cathedral in Garden Grove, California. I first heard about Anderson from Bill Blair. "He's a real warrior," Bill told me. "The kind of guy you'd want with you in a foxhole." Serious praise from Bill Blair, the man with whom I had formed what Anderson would call "a healing partnership." We all need foxhole friends.

Diagnosed with metastasized lung cancer in 1984, Anderson was given thirty days to live. Refusing to accept his terminal prognosis, he made a decision to do all he could to triumph over his cancer. As I write, Anderson is alive and well and has published several powerful and hope-filled books sharing his own experience, and presenting a "road map to recovery" based on his interviews with over 19,000 "cancer conquerors." I carry his book, *Cancer: 50 Essential Things to Do*, in my duffel bag when I travel. (The best way I know to introduce people to a valuable book is to let them hold it in their hands.) Anderson has provided us with a state-of-the-art conquerers' handbook. I strongly recommend that you go to his Web site, www.cancerrecovery.org, click on Foundation for Cancer Research and Wellness, and check out the Pyramid.

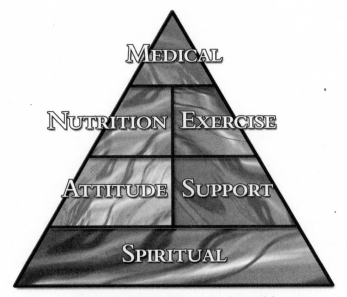

Figure 2. Cancer Recovery Pyramid

If you click on ATTITUDE, you will find "The Cancer Conqueror's Ten Key Beliefs," a summary of the core survival beliefs of cancer patients who lived when they were supposed to have died. Anderson opens with the words: "I Believe . . ." What follows is a cancer conqueror's rendition of the Apostle's Creed:

> *I believe I become a cancer conqueror*
> *Not because I go into remission*
> *But because I become a new person.*

I have to tell you that, in accord with the overall military metaphor of "blockade," "surveillance" and "fighting cancer," my Refusenik self far prefers the notion of being a "cancer conqueror" — or as Colin Powell says, a "cancer warrior" — to that of being merely a "survivor."

To borrow a phrase from Bette Davis, the lifestyle therapy Anderson recommends "ain't for sissies." It requires that you possess *"the unshakable belief that recovery is possible, available, and that you can be the agent of that recovery."* I can put a check mark next to that one. And yet, when I consider the hard work, dedication and self-discipline involved in lifestyle therapy, I understand why most men prefer to rely solely on conventional treatments for prostate cancer.

These days, as I continue to make my way through the medical mine-field, I confess that I regularly fall short in following much of Anderson's sound advice. But where I do keep the faith is by sending my immune system what is, for me, the ultimate Emotional-Chemical Text Message, and it is this: *My cancer is reversible, and I am healing my life.*

"IMMUNE SYSTEM YOGA" FOR REFUSENIKS

A batch of studies now claim that visualizing your exercise routine gives you at least some of the benefits of actually logging time in the gym. You can increase your metabolic rate — and that means you burn calories — by sim-ply *visualizing* yourself on the treadmill or working out with weights. And that's just for openers. This capacity for psycho-physical self-regulation has many levels. Move the bar up a notch and there's your champion golfer shooting an eagle *in his mind* on the fourteenth hole at Muirfield and then stepping up to the tee and actually making the shots. Brain scans show that when you imagine an event, the same areas of the brain light up as during the actual event. Apparently the brain doesn't distinguish between a vivid mental experience and an actual physical one.

Move the bar up another notch and you can be taught meditative techniques that enable you to raise the temperature of your hands just by focusing your attention on your palms and imagining them getting warm. People experienced in meditation can change their heart rates and control pain and bleeding, which means that we have the ability to control our bodies right down to the cellular level.

VISUALIZATION FOR HEALING CANCER

During the 2010 Olympics, there were several references to skiers who were "big on visualization," with the announcer explaining, "You see yourself crossing the finish line, and the mechanics fall into place." Athletes seem to be leading the way in making visualization popular. And yet since the early 1970s, O. Carl Simonton, MD, the first Western practitioner to link mind and emotions to the immune system, has been teaching his patients to use imaging techniques to fight cancer. His original concept, based on the old video game in which Pac-Men gobbled up the "bad guys" to win the game, was of little Pac-Men destroying the cancer cells.* This may seem like a stretch, but since he began using imagery, Dr. Simonton has trained thousands of health care professionals in his very successful methods.

The way people image is as varied as their fingerprints. Some people see their tumor being shredded by sharp-beaked birds or torn to bits by ravenous black leopards. Others simply picture the tumor shrinking, or visualize it as a block of ice and melt it with light descending from heaven. Imaging doesn't have to be anatomically correct. It's whatever works for you. And a host of anecdotal evidence supports the fact that if you persevere, imaging *does* work. There are even studies showing that people who pictured little men carrying calcium bricks to rebuild their broken arms actually healed nearly 50% faster than those who didn't visualize.

---

*In his 1978 book *Getting Well Again*, Dr. Simonton describes the body's white blood cells as tiny Pac-Men "swarming over the cancer cells, picking up and carrying off the dead and dying ones, flushing them out of the body through the liver and kidneys."

Since I am not all that good at visualizing, I found a picture (see below) of a cancer cell under attack by killer T cells dispatched by the immune system. I had the picture enlarged and taped it to the wall in front of my computer screen. Now, each time I look up from my keyboard, there it is—the "enemy"—being blasted by my own personal Star Wars battle force.

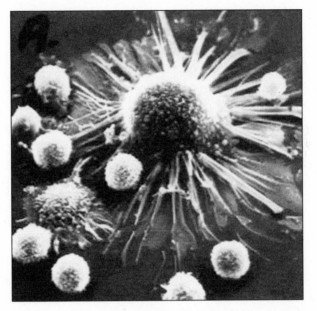

Image 4. Cancer cell under attack by the immune system.

If the idea of visualization is new to you, there are dozens of prerecorded guided imagery tapes available that can help you get into the relaxed, focused state required for successful imaging. I urge you to check it out because at the very least, the general feeling of peacefulness evoked by the meditative state reduces your level of stress and anxiety, and that alone enhances your immune function.

LAUGHTER: THE BEST MEDICINE

"The best doctors in the world are Doctor Diet, Doctor Quiet and Doctor Merryman." So wrote Jonathan Swift (1667–1743). Without a doubt, my favorite of the three is Doctor Merryman. Perhaps you have heard it said that God's favorite music is laughter. I concur.

Laughter is the ultimate antioxidant. Here's how the Discovery Health Web site describes the impact of laughter on the immune system: "When we laugh, natural killer cells which destroy tumors and viruses increase, along with Gamma-interferon (a disease-fighting protein), T cells (important for our immune system) and B-cells (which make disease-fighting antibodies). As well as lowering blood pressure, laughter increases oxygen in the blood, which also encourages healing." So whatever other supplements you take, be sure to include laughter.

Believe me when I say that my somewhat warped sense of humor has been a blessing to me in devastating moments. Time and again I have seen the relief and release that even stupid jokes or bawdy humor can provide to men who are under the gun. In his book *Anatomy of an Illness*, Norman Cousins calls laughter "internal jogging," and recommends a healing diet whose main course is laughter seasoned with liberal lashings of vitamin C. Cousins laughed his way back to health with old Groucho movies. For me, it was the amazing Carol Burnett.

I wasn't expecting it, but she made me laugh. Oh how she made me laugh! As I replay her shows, particularly her specials, I can actually feel myself getting healthier. My immune system knows that for me, this is the real McCoy. Her humor is physical. It's cerebral. It's fall-down slapstick. It's luminous! Thank you, Carol Burnett. I'm so glad we spent this time together.

So find what works for you, because studies have shown that the relaxation response following a good laugh lasts at least forty-five minutes. The message is clear: *Lighten up!*

A FINAL WORD ON ROMANCING YOUR IMMUNE SYSTEM

It was a starry night in the islands, and I was sitting with my friend Martin Rayner on the deck of his schooner, anchored in Manele Bay. I remember him patiently listening as I enumerated all the problems I was facing, all my difficulties and woes. He let me talk without interrupting, just nodding and smiling sympathetically until I had run my litany of complaints. When I finally asked, "So, what do you think I ought to do?" Martin reached out, patted my arm and said, "Have a good time. Have a good time, and make sure that everyone around you is having a good time."

These days, for the sake of my immune system, I do my best to avoid stressful situations, try to eat well, complain rarely, laugh a lot, send mostly jolly Emotional-Chemical Text Messages and, yes, as far as it's within my ability to do so, follow Martin Rayner's wise counsel.

THE DOCTOR'S VIEW

Ralph's title for this chapter is very appropriate. The start of our "courtship" of the immune system is lost in the mists of time. Around three thousand years ago, King Solomon declared that "a joyful heart is good medicine, but a broken spirit dries up the bones." The "wet" part of the bones, otherwise known as the marrow, is where the immune system is located. I don't know where Solomon got his understanding but the message is clear. When facing a major health challenge, ignoring the importance of thought, lifestyle or belief system is a big mistake. Modern interest in pursuing this courtship has given rise to disciplines as sophisticated as psychoneuroimmunology. Ralph's take on the entire mind–body interaction is an original and positive contribution to this field of study.

22.

HOW PROSTATE CANCER
CAN MAKE YOU LIVE LONGER:
GETTING TO THE DOCTOR'S OFFICE

Good habits are as addictive as bad habits, and a lot more rewarding.

— HARVEY MACKAY

I am often struck by the prodigious efforts men make to get the best treatment for prostate cancer while totally ignoring other diseases that are more deadly. I'll never forget the unexpected phone call I received from the distraught wife of a fifty-five-year-old patient who had consulted me about prostate cancer only a week earlier. Her first anguished words were, "How did you know?" Initially I was confused. "How did I know what?" I responded. "How did you know that my husband had heart disease?"

At first I didn't even understand what she was talking about. Then she told me her husband had died in his sleep from a massive heart attack just four days after our consultation. She was referring to the advice I had given him during the consultation—that he should get checked for heart disease. There was no indication of a heart problem. I was just following my standard screening routine.

Deeply sorry for her loss, I explained to her that when men come to my office, they are profoundly concerned about dying from prostate cancer. However, most have *Low-Risk* variants of the disease that are practically never fatal. Therefore, simply because they are average American males, their risk from a heart attack is much greater than the risk of dying from prostate cancer. This is why I routinely recommend cardiac screening, even though most men protest by telling me what excellent shape they are in, how their cholesterol is low, and how good they feel generally. I argue that a straightforward look at the common causes of death in men suggests that screening for heart disease makes sense (Table 7).

Table 7: Annual Death Rates in Men

Heart Disease	350,000
Lung Cancer	89,000
Stroke	65,000
Accidents	63,000
Emphysema	62,000
Diabetes	31,000
Prostate Cancer	**27,000**
Flu/Pneumonia	27,000
Colon Cancer	25,000

PROSTATE CANCER IS THE SPUR

Screening for health problems is not very popular. It can be inconvenient, uncomfortable and, on occasion, expensive, as insurance companies do not always pay for scanning procedures (see below). What's more, screening can lead to false positive results, causing additional stress and concern. Despite all these drawbacks, screening is our best defense and the only tool available for early detection of certain common and preventable problems. However, even prior to obtaining body scans, a simple and relatively inexpensive first step is to obtain some routine blood tests (Table 8).

Table 8: Routine Blood Tests

Panel	Function
Basic Metabolic	Kidney function and mineral levels
Hepatic	Liver and nutritional status
CBC	Anemia, immune function and clotting
Lipid	LDL and HDL (good and bad cholesterol)
Vitamin B12, D	Deficiencies are common
Thyroid	Controls metabolic activity

These tests are relatively inexpensive and widely available at almost any lab, doctor's office or hospital. Abnormal results can signal significant underlying health problems like diabetes, liver disease, kidney disease, vitamin deficiencies or hormonal imbalances. All of these problems are much easier to treat when they are detected early. For example, low vitamin B12 levels can cause memory problems and can occur despite taking B12 supplements because as we get older our gastrointestinal tract absorbs B12 less efficiently. When detected, this deficiency can easily be corrected with B12 preparations that melt under the tongue and are absorbed into the blood directly through the mucus membranes of the mouth.

SCANNING THE HEART TO MEASURE CORONARY PLAQUE

One of the most significant advances for detecting heart disease has been the refinement of a body scanning technique called computerized tomography, commonly referred to as CT scans. Body scans have been around for some years, but improving technology now offers substantially better information about the inner workings of the body. If we use the analogy of a camera, the older scans could not take pictures of the moving parts of the body because they had such slow exposure times. Images of moving organs like the heart, the lungs and the colon always came out blurred. Today, however, we achieve excellent image quality.

I am not advocating that total body scans be undertaken willy-nilly. The value of global body scanning is highly debatable because random scanning frequently uncovers minor abnormalities that require stressful, time-consuming and expensive testing and lead to further scans, blood tests, consultations, biopsies or even surgery, just to prove that the suspicious area is not the beginning of some malignant process.

There are, however, valid uses for CT scans. Detecting cholesterol plaque in the coronary arteries is one such legitimate use. Because they tend to be older, men with prostate cancer are also at high risk for developing atherosclerotic plaque, otherwise known as hardening of the arteries. Plaque can build up to the point where an artery is totally blocked, causing a heart attack or stroke. Over 400,000 men in the United States die of either heart attack or stroke every year, and twice that many men suffer nonfatal strokes and heart attacks. Atherosclerosis is a silent disease until a major event occurs. *One-third of initial heart attacks are fatal.* Some experts recommend relying on cholesterol testing to detect which men have more plaque; however, those tests are often imprecise. Some men with high cholesterol levels have minimal plaque whereas others with low cholesterol have extensive plaque. With something as dangerous as heart disease, there is no room for guesswork or for error.

Fast CT scans accurately evaluate the status of the coronary arteries by indicating how much plaque is present. Of course since average Americans are dying of heart attacks in droves, even having an average amount of plaque is serious. The checklist below outlines necessary steps men should take if they have an average or above average amount of plaque:

What You Do if Excess Plaque Is Discovered

See a qualified cardiologist
Obtain a cardiac stress test annually
Obtain an ultrasound of the carotid arteries
Start a statin drug such as Lipitor or Crestor
Start aspirin 81 mg a day (if there are no contraindications to aspirin)
Reduce blood pressure to 125 over 75
Diet and exercise

With heart attacks at epidemic levels, it seems foolish to forgo a simple ten-minute, $300 scan to find out the status of one's arteries. Repeat scans should probably be done every three to five years to determine if the plaque is progressing or regressing. Some people express concern about excess radiation exposure, but fortunately state-of-the-art scanners have been developed that minimize radiation dose. Present technology has reduced the radiation dose from a heart scan down to the same exposure you get with a set of dental x-rays.

OSTEOPOROSIS

Osteoporosis is defined as weakened bone from loss of calcium. Fractures can occur in the spine, rib, wrist and hip. The process is completely silent up to the point of a fracture. Compression fractures of the spine can be extremely painful, result in loss of height and, when advanced, result in a forward curvature of the spine known as the "dowager's hump." All such fractures are associated with decreased survival.[1]

Osteoporosis is mistakenly thought to occur only in women, but fully a third of all hip fractures occur in men. There are many causes. Men who are slender have less bone reserve and are more predisposed to osteoporosis. Thyroid or parathyroid hyperactivity can also contribute to osteoporosis. Other causes are excessive use of alcohol, caffeine or tobacco.

Cortisone, used to treat asthma or arthritis, is another common culprit. Excess vitamin A has also been associated with osteoporosis and fractures.[2] Lack of exercise, lack of sunlight exposure (low vitamin D) and low calcium intake are additional potential causes, and unless precautions are taken, bone fractures can occur more frequently in men treated with TIP.[3,4]

Osteoporosis is detected by scanning. However, some scans are less accurate than others. In my opinion the DEXA scan underestimates osteoporosis in men. The problem with DEXA is that men over age fifty have much more calcified degenerative arthritis of the lower back than women. The excess calcium surrounding the spine causes the DEXA scan to read artificially high, masking the presence of osteoporosis. For men a more accurate technique called quantitative CAT scan, or QCT, is preferable. QCT accurately measures calcium density in the center of the vertebral column. Many health care providers are unaware of the DEXA scan's limitations even though these limitations have been well documented in a study from Massachusetts General Hospital.[5] In this study, forty-one men at an average age of sixty-eight underwent both DEXA and QCT scanning. QCT detected preexisting osteoporosis in 63% whereas DEXA only detected it in 5%.

Checklist for Treatment of Osteoporosis

Calcium citrate 500 mg with dinner and at bedtime
Vitamin D 2000 IU daily (or check blood levels and adjust dose accordingly)
A monthly pill such as Actonel or Boniva
Exercise (preferably some form of weight lifting)
Repeat bone density testing every two years to ensure treatment is working

---

COLON CANCER

Colon cancer kills about the same number of men in the United States each year as prostate cancer. Unfortunately, having prostate cancer does not provide immunity from colon cancer. Back in the 1990s, when chemotherapy was just coming into its own, I was consulted by Peter Lenning, who had advanced prostate cancer and bone metastasis. In the six months prior to seeing me his PSA had risen from less than 50 to over 1000! Fortunately I had just heard about a new chemotherapy drug from some researchers at USC in a clinic where I volunteered. The doctors there were excited about a lung cancer patient whose bone metastasis melted away when he was treated with Taxotere. When I heard "bone metastasis" I naturally thought of my advanced prostate cancer patient with the same affliction. Peter had relatively few options so he gave Taxotere a try. Over the next six months his PSA miraculously dropped from over 1000 to less than 1. Obviously we were thrilled. After a year we stopped the treatment. Slowly his PSA started to creep up, but only at a snail's pace.

On Peter's first visit to our office, well before his first Taxotere treatment, his physical examination showed some blood in his stool. We advised further evaluation with a colonoscopy. Despite repeated admonitions Peter never seemed to get around to having it done. A year later he was still procrastinating. He even had an overt episode of rectal bleeding. Finally, two years later, a more severe occurrence of bleeding convinced him to get a checkup. By then it was too late. The colon cancer had already metastasized. Peter died about a year later—from colon cancer. At that time he had been off Taxotere for two years. His PSA was only 6.

Colonoscopy detects colon cancer when it is in the polyp stage, long before it spreads. Screening should never be delayed until rectal bleeding occurs. Colonoscopy needs to be done every ten years starting at age fifty. Alternatively, a scanning methodology using a CT—a virtual colonoscopy—can be used. There are advantages and disadvantages of both approaches. With virtual colonoscopy there is no need for sedation and practically no risk of a colon perforation. However, virtual colonoscopy may not be quite as accurate as a regular colonoscopy. If a polyp is detected on a virtual colonoscopy, a regular colonoscopy is needed to remove it. Whichever method is used, colon cancer deaths can be almost eliminated with screening.

SARCOPENIA

Studies prove that strength equates with health and youthfulness. To most of us, weakness is synonymous with being old. Yet muscle loss is a natural result of aging. Sarcopenia—the technical word for low muscle mass—has a very negative effect on health. In a study published in 2002 in the *New England Journal of Medicine* the effect of fitness on survival was evaluated in 2,500 healthy men and women with an average age of fifty-five. Fitness was measured via a standard treadmill test. After the treadmill the participants were allocated into three groups of varying fitness: the strong, the average and the weak. To determine survival after ten years, the researchers queried the social security data base to determine who was still collecting a check—they figured that only dead people fail to collect a check! They found that 90% of the strong, 75% of the average and only 60% of the weak were still alive. The impact of improved fitness on longevity was so great that *physically fit smokers outlived the nonsmokers who had poor physical conditioning.*

The best way to build muscle is with weight training. As previously discussed, for men on TIP the risk of muscle loss is even more critical. Without regular weight training, men on TIP lose muscle mass quickly.[7] Strength training has to be intense enough to produce muscle failure— lifting weights to the point of no longer being able to lift. Muscle failure sends a clear signal to the muscle that it is inadequate so that further muscle growth is necessary. A typical program requires two or three one-hour sessions each week. During a one-hour session, all the major muscle groups of the body are exercised with three sets of ten to twelve repetitions. When men closely adhere to this recommended protocol, the impact of tiredness and weakness from TIP is almost totally eliminated. Obviously, men with normal testosterone levels who are not on TIP experience an even greater enhancement of their energy levels.

LUNG CANCER

Early diagnosis of lung cancer is vital, as it is almost universally fatal when diagnosed after symptoms such as cough, chest pain or weight loss occur. When symptoms are present the average survival is only nine months. Fortunately, fast CT scans can detect early stage lung cancers when they are still treatable. Surgeons use a telescopic device called thoracoscopy to remove the cancer. (This is very similar to laparoscopy for operations in the abdominal area.) Cure rates for men with lung cancers detected by screening are often as high as 80%. Active smokers and those with a significant smoking history who have stopped smoking in the last fifteen years should have a lung scan done annually.

BLADDER CANCER AND MELANOMA

Bladder cancer kills about 6,000 men each year, five times less than prostate cancer. Early diagnosis, as is the case with most cancers, is the best way to reduce mortality rates. Early bladder cancer is often signaled by the presence of microscopic blood in the urine, which can be detected with a urine analysis, a simple test that should be a standard part of the general annual physical examination.

Melanoma is a cancer in which fatal cases are half as common as those of bladder cancer. Three thousand men die each year from melanoma, a pigmented cancer that looks like a new mole in its early stages. When melanoma spreads there are very few effective methods of treatment. It needs to be diagnosed and treated at the earliest possible stage. If detected early, it is usually curable with surgical removal. An annual visit to the dermatologist can save your life.

OTHER CAUSES

The next most common killers after prostate cancer and colon cancer are flu and pneumonia. Although most people know about flu vaccines, many are unaware of FDA-approved antibiotics like Tamiflu and Flumadine. To be effective these antibiotics need to be started promptly after the onset of symptoms. They can also be used to prevent illness in healthy family members who have been exposed. The classic symptoms of flu are fever, body aches and severe sore throat. Unfortunately, these antibiotics do not work against other viruses like the common cold. Sadly, patients have been brainwashed with the mistaken belief that antibiotics work for bacteria but not for viruses. So when the flu strikes, no one thinks to call the doctor to get a prescription for Tamiflu which, if started within twenty-four hours, rapidly relieves flu symptoms.

Another sensible preventative measure is often overlooked—getting a vaccine against pneumonia. Pneumovax is administered every five years and is recommended for people over sixty-five and for people of any age with chronic conditions like asthma, emphysema or heart disease.

CONCLUSION

Certain potentially life-threatening illnesses can be detected at an earlier, more treatable stage by making an annual visit to the doctor's office for evaluation. It takes a lot to motivate us guys to go see a doctor, but a diagnosis of prostate cancer seems to do the trick. Often for the first time in a man's life a relationship with a doctor is established and an opportunity is created for discussion about other common and preventable diseases. Trying to detect every possible illness is impractical, and many illnesses are too uncommon to justify screening. However, looking for common preventable conditions like heart disease, colon cancer and osteoporosis makes sense.

Heart disease is widespread and much can be done to reduce mortality. Over the last fifteen years, deaths from heart attacks have been reduced by 50% due to dietary changes, treating high cholesterol and earlier detection. The risk of dying from colon cancer can be almost eliminated by simply doing a screening colonoscopy every ten years. Early cancers in the form of polyps are simply removed during the screening process. Osteoporosis is detectable with a simple scan, and treatment can be as easy as taking a single monthly pill. Certainly, if it's worth taking the considerable time necessary to treat a low-grade illness like prostate cancer, it also makes sense to invest the relatively small amount of time and effort it takes to ensure that these other common and potentially serious conditions are prevented.

THE PATIENT'S VIEW

Dozens of men I have interviewed have stated emphatically that, if it hadn't been for their having prostate cancer, they might never have gotten the checkups they needed. They discovered clogged arteries, osteoporosis, liver problems and on and on. So maybe thanks to prostate cancer, and the checkups we get as a result of that diagnosis, many of us will not die at the hand of some killer we never even realized was stalking us.

23.

BY WAY OF SUMMING UP

We live in a time when there are more techniques for healing than ever
before. The question we must ask is this: What is it, beyond or beneath
these techniques, that really fosters the healing process?

—O. CARL SIMONTON, MD, *Healers on Healing, "The Harmony of Health"*

At this point I feel like the Ancient Mariner of Prostate Cancer, tugging at
your sleeve and saying, "Just one more thing," and "Here's something that
really helped me; it might be useful for you . . ." If I had to describe my
journey in ten simple words, I would say this: *I have come to regard prostate
cancer as my teacher.*

Had I known, when I was first diagnosed, all the things I have learned
during my two decades of living—actually *coexisting*—with this disease, I
would have started much sooner to use what I have learned, not only to
help heal the cancer but also to heal my life.

STATUS REPORT

I was fifty-eight when I first went to Jeff Harris for a checkup, and back then,
in 1990, the prostate cancer field was still in what Bill Blair called "the iron
lung period." So by not submitting to a second biopsy for nine years, and
not rushing into surgery or unfocused radiation—the only two treatment
options available at that time—I dodged some major bullets. My reasoning
may have been suspect. Reasoning is not high on a Refusenik's list of good
qualities. But it appears my instincts were sound, and my decision to protect
my quality of life by avoiding radical invasive treatment has paid off.

Now, at seventy-eight, I still have options. After all these years I am still
in the process of decision making. I can continue this journey, continue to
watch and wait and monitor the cancer. Or I can go for one of the more
sophisticated treatments available today.

When I last discussed my options with Mark, he reminded me that the way the cancer has been behaving over the past twenty years is reassuring.

"How the cancer behaves is the most important predictor," Mark told me. "It supersedes Gleason score, it supersedes stage and PSA. Those indicators are all ways to try to predict how the cancer will behave. In your case, Ralph, we've had two decades to observe its behavior, and that behavior has to trump all the stats. Once you identify a behavior pattern, you need to allow that valuable information to percolate into the decision-making process. Despite a Gleason 3 + 4 and seminal vesicle involvement, after the Combidex showed no cancer in the lymph nodes, it doesn't seem quite so Looney Tunes for you to still be monitoring it."

In Mark's experience, cancers do not tend to change their stripes after twenty years. "It's like having new neighbors," he said. "With time you learn that they keep their property neat, that their dog won't crap on your lawn and that if you want to borrow a cup of sugar, sugar is what you'll get. Well, the same with prostate cancer."

So Mark is not pushing me to go for treatment. And Jeanne has always supported my decisions. Still, I am in uncharted waters. Tell my stats to a roomful of surgeons or radiation oncologists, and the chorus will be a resounding "Treat it!"

There's no way I can prove them wrong, no way I want to argue the case at this point. And yet there is one other thing influencing me to continue monitoring my situation, and that is Duke Bahn's recent color Doppler ultrasound, in which there appears to still be no blood flow to the tumor. I take this as a good sign.

The way I see my medical situation now, I have three choices: I could go back on some form of TIP, maybe Casodex alone, or possibly add the "immune cocktail" that Mark describes in chapter 24. Or I could go for a cure with IMRT. Or I can continue active surveillance and wait for one of the promising new treatments already in the pipeline. So although I have lived with prostate cancer for two decades, I am still in the same unresolved decision-making mode as the guy who has just been diagnosed. And I still have to deal with the same fears.

TIMOR MORTIS CONTURBAT ME

When I wake in the night, sweating, panicked, terrified I'm going to die of this disease, I think of the Latin response from the medieval Office of the Dead, the Third Nocturn of Matins. *Timor mortis conturbat me*: "Fear of death riles me up." Every time my PSA or Gleason hikes up, every time my status changes, I am swamped again by the fear that I might have tempted fate one too many times by failing to act, by not going for a cure. When the fear becomes overwhelming, I pick up the phone and call one of my foxhole buddies. Talking with a guy who has been there, done that does a lot to diffuse the worst panic. It also helps that I've lived through this fear many times before. The important thing is not to let fear stampede you into making treatment decisions you might live to regret.

Fear is an untrustworthy advisor.

Once you are diagnosed with prostate cancer there is always the possibility—even if you go for a cure—that the cancer will return. There are no guarantees. Which is why, in "The Patient's Track," I have stressed the value of faith, a positive attitude and the things we can do to help ourselves. As Greg Anderson says: "Retaining a medical team without doing all you can to help yourself is like attempting to walk with one stilt."

SEVEN HEALING PRACTICES

After coming this far with me on my journey, if you belong to the "Tortoise Clan" of prostate cancers, I hope it makes sense to you to consider coexisting with this cancer, rather than surrendering to radical, invasive treatment. With this in mind, I want to share with you some of the nonmedical practices I am convinced have contributed to keeping my cancer in check and to my overall quality of life all these years:

- I laugh a lot more than I used to before I understood the healing power of laughter. For me, laughter is the ultimate antioxidant.
- I have become a big fan of gratitude. Part of my daily routine is to be mindful of how grateful I am to all the people who have supported me on my prostate cancer journey, how grateful I am, in fact, for everything in my life, even the simple miracle of turning on a tap and having clean water to drink.
- Remembering Deepak Chopra's words, "Every cell in your body is eavesdropping on your thoughts," I do my best to let go of toxic thinking and emotions that are a drain on my immune system.
- To the best of my ability, I stay in the present, letting go of past grievances and regrets, refusing to squander energy worrying about the future.

- I put my faith, my love of God, into action by making service to others part of my own healing. It is no coincidence that volunteers live longer.

- I find time to play, to stroll on the beach, listen to music, reconnect with old friends. I make time for activities that delight my soul and nourish my spirit.

- I work on the projects that will come after this book; I make plans for what I want to do with the rest of my long life.

These common sense, mundane practices have enriched my life on this long and challenging journey.

And there is one other thing I do. When a man calls me in a panic, having just received a death sentence, I always give him my friend Harvey's advice: *No matter how bad your cancer gets, never listen to the naysayers. Someone has survived it, someone who had it that bad before you. If the doctors say your odds of making it through five months—let alone five years—are one in a hundred, don't look at what the ninety-nine did, because that didn't work and it isn't for you. Find the one who made it through and imitate him.*

ENDGAME

Not long ago, I attended a dinner meeting of the Prostate Cancer Club, at which an assortment of oncologists, surgeons and radiation specialists dine together and read and discuss their recently published scientific papers. These monthly gatherings are held in the Milken Building in Santa Monica, headquarters of the Prostate Cancer Foundation (PCF).

After being diagnosed with advanced prostate cancer in 1993 and given twelve months to live, billionaire buccaneer Michael Milken survived and founded PCF, now the world's leading organization for funding prostate cancer research. That evening, during dinner, Milken dropped by long enough to say a few encouraging words—and to predict that prostate cancer will be history by 2016. Well, nobody has done more to make that happen. I can only say: *From Michael Milken's mouth to God's ears!*

On December 12, 2004, a foggy Saturday in Marina del Rey, when Mark and I first sat down to work on the proposal for this book, Mark said, "Let's pray." Ever since that day, before we started to work, we'd pray— pray that our book would be acceptable to our publisher, of service to many and pleasing in God's sight.

I have come to understand how strong a remedy is faith in the loving presence of the Divine. I regard my faith as the ultimate ℞ from the Master Compounding Chemist, enabling me to live successfully with this cancer for over twenty years.

And I am grateful for so many things. I give thanks that I am blessed with the chronic form of this disease, the tortoise of prostate cancers. I give thanks that I can wait, and while I wait I still toss back my daily jigger of the APeX Solution, along with my Avodart and aspirin. And I am grateful that the Duke's color Doppler images still show no new blood flow to the tumor.

I will continue to seek out unusual remedies that are found beneath the medical radar—the latest and most promising being the "energy tools" developed by Dr. Yury Kronn. So stay tuned in. The quest goes on.

As for the Enchanted Shotgun itself? Elusive as it remains, I have indeed caught glimpses of it by moonlight. And I can tell you this much: It is double-barreled, and hope and faith are its triggers.

So what would we like you to come away with after reading this book? First, a feeling that the promise made on the cover is being kept: that the "invasion" is being repulsed. That increasing emphasis is being placed on quality of life. That we will continue to see a steady decline in *unnecessary everything*—biopsies, invasive treatment and all forms of collateral damage. And finally, that working together, Mark and I have accomplished what we set out to do—write a book that informs you, entertains you, calms your fears and leaves you with good reasons for hope.

THE DOCTOR'S VIEW

My writing partner is a pioneer. During the years he stuck with his go-slow strategy—staying on active surveillance and then opting for TIP—the technology progressed far more rapidly than his cancer. If you are newly diagnosed, the good news is that advances over the next five years are expected to be more significant than anything we have seen in the last twenty.

So the message is the same, only stronger. When it's appropriate, wait and go slow. Use the time to educate yourself about the disease, the doctors and your priorities. You will know that you are on the right path when, like Ralph, you are able to view your prostate cancer experience as a teaching.

24.

GENUINE HOPE FOR MEN WITH RELAPSED DISEASE

There is one thing that gives radiance to everything. It is the idea of something just around the corner.

— G. K. CHESTERTON

Cure is the goal of surgery and radiation. But after treatment, men face a five-year incubation period, waiting to see if the cancer will return. Relapses are common, occurring in about a third of men who undergo surgery or radiation. Doctor visits for checkups and PSA testing generate substantial anxiety because a cancer relapse is first signaled by a rise in PSA. However, most men are poorly informed. They wrongly assume that, like other cancers, a relapse is imminently life threatening. Fortunately, the large majority are not fatal, and long survival is the norm.

One of the reasons the return of prostate cancer is far less serious compared to other types of cancer is because PSA testing signals a relapse when the disease is still microscopic, far too small to be seen on scans. Early treatment of minimal disease is much more effective than trying to control advanced disease. Unfortunately, other types of cancer are usually detected at a more advanced stage, when they become visible on radiographic scans.

Therefore, with relapsed prostate cancer the theme once again is selecting treatment based on quality of life. Given the variety of new drugs and treatments and new ways of thinking about these available options, relapsed disease can be effectively controlled with far fewer side effects than in the past.

NEW WAYS OF PRESCRIBING TIP—LESS IS MORE

Relapsed prostate cancer responds extremely well to TIP, resulting in remissions that average more than ten years.[1] With such effective therapy, many doctors leave their relapsed patients on TIP indefinitely. They are reluctant to discontinue TIP because of the fear that control of the cancer will be lost. However, as we have seen previously in this book, long-term TIP has undesirable side effects.

In the 1990s, concerned with improving quality of life for our patients on TIP, my former partner, Stephen Strum, and I started using an approach that is now called *intermittent therapy*—providing patients with regular holidays from TIP.[2] Back then, stopping TIP was considered radical. Today, after the publication of two randomized prospective trials,[3,4] many specialists have concluded that intermittent therapy is both safe and effective.[5,6] Furthermore, Dr. Strum and I reported in the 2006 *Journal of Urology* that administering Proscar delays cancer growth, *doubling* the length of the holiday period and allowing men to maintain normal testosterone levels, increased energy and a restored libido.[2] Not surprisingly, men are grateful for the opportunity to remain off treatment for a longer period, as Ralph has done. In our daily practice, using Proscar (see Appendix) during the TIP holiday is now standard. The early detection of relapse and the intermittent use of TIP mean that relapsed cancer can be treated more like a chronic condition rather than a life-threatening illness.

NEW DRUGS JUST OVER THE HORIZON

After many years, men with relapsed disease who have been taking TIP either continuously or intermittently may face a rising PSA despite ongoing use of TIP. Until recently, it was assumed that resistance to TIP was caused by mutated cancer cells, cells able to grow in an environment devoid of testosterone. Now we know that this assumption was wrong. Resistant cells still need testosterone to survive and proliferate. They are able to proliferate despite low levels of testosterone in the blood because they learn to manufacture their own testosterone. Armed with this new insight, researchers have designed medicines to counteract these maverick cancer cells by blocking testosterone synthesis.

A new drug, Abiraterone, developed by Cougar Biotechnology, is one fruit of such research. Trials show that Abiraterone induces a significant decline in PSA in 70% of men with TIP resistance. As of early 2010 a phase III trial of over a thousand men is now under way. We hope that the FDA will release this medication in 2011. Other companies besides

Cougar are also working to improve the way testosterone is blocked inside the cancer cell. A San Francisco company, Medivation, has developed a promising, more potent androgen receptor antagonist called MDV 3100 that works like a supercharged form of Casodex. A large phase III trial aimed at getting FDA approval for this drug was initiated in July 2009.

NEW THINKING ABOUT RADIATION

Besides TIP, radiation is the other commonly used treatment for relapse after surgery. Most often, radiation is directed to the prostatic fossa (prostate bed) to treat microscopic disease left behind after the operation. Broadening the fields to encompass the adjacent lymph nodes was discouraged in the past because of the risk of permanent radiation damage to the nearby intestines. Also, cancer experts used to believe that metastasis in the lymph nodes always meant the disease had spread to other parts of the body as well, and that it was incurable. We now know that exceptions to this belief are common. Radiation treatment directed at metastatic disease in the lymph nodes of the pelvis may still be curative.[7,8] And now, with the flexibility of IMRT and careful targeting, the risk of bowel damage from radiation is greatly reduced.[9]

Bob Doherty, a sixty-one-year-old travel consultant, benefited greatly from IMRT to the lymph nodes. When he first relapsed after surgery he initially controlled his disease for many years with intermittent TIP. But in late 2006 he had a Combidex scan in Holland showing three cancerous lymph nodes in the right pelvis and one in the left pelvis, all of which were treated with IMRT. In mid-2009, now off TIP for more than 3 years, he continues to have a low and stable PSA at less than 0.01 with normal testosterone levels.

New research is showing that radiation kills cancer in a manner quite different from what was previously believed. Whereas radiation does destroy some of the cancer cells by disrupting cellular DNA, it also increases immune activity against the cancer. This increased immune activity occurs in two ways. First, it disrupts cell architecture, exposing previously hidden cancer cell proteins to the immune system, enabling the immune system "to get the scent and go on the attack." Second, radiation kills off traitorous regulatory immune cells (the T_{Reg} cells), a component of our immune systems that paradoxically works in partnership *with* the cancer, shielding the disease from immune attack. Radiation in essence uncloaks the cancer cells by killing off the T_{Reg} cell "cover."

NEW HOPE FOR A CURE THROUGH IMMUNE THERAPY

Utilizing the immune system to fight cancer is a rapidly advancing area of research and new drug development. The immune system, as it relates to fighting cancer, is made up of three components: 1) the killer cells, 2) the regulatory T_{Reg} cells and 3) the dendritic cells that provide a "scent" to the killer cells enabling them to better home in on the cancer. Enhancing dendritic cell activity is the mechanism of action for the recently FDA-approved cancer treatment called Provenge.

For years, attempts to stimulate the immune system to attack cancer have fallen short because they failed to deal with the T_{Reg} cells. T_{Reg} cells, operating in their normal role, police the immune system to ensure that the killer cells don't get out of hand and attack healthy tissue; they are our protection from diseases of overactive immunity such as lupus and multiple sclerosis. However, they can blunt cancer therapies designed to work by stimulating the immune system.

Research now shows that cancer cells can exploit and distort the function of the T_{Reg} cells. The cancer "kidnaps" this regulatory component of the immune system by using the T_{Reg} cells to blunt killer cell activity and also to increase other immunosuppressive hormones like vascular endothelial growth factor (VEGF) and transforming growth factor beta (TGF-Beta). The cancer cells recruit T_{Reg} cells and use them as a shield against the killer cells. This new understanding finally explains why the immune system fails to attack the cancer. Immune inactivity is not a *weakness* of the immune system; it is a type of *blindness*.

Unequivocal evidence for immune-mediated PSA responses in men with relapsed disease first came to my attention in June 2006 when Doctors Brian Rini and Eric Small reported in the *Journal of Urology* that remissions *lasting more than five years* occurred in 25% of the men they treated with Leukine.[10] Leukine, otherwise known by the ponderous name granulocyte-macrophage colony-stimulating factor or GM-CSF, is approved by the FDA to stimulate the rapid growth of a type of white blood cells called granulocytes, the immune cells that fight bacteria. However, Leukine was subsequently found to have an additional favorable effect on the immune system, that of stimulating dendritic cells, the immune cells that function to identify cancer cells and stimulate the killer cells to attack them.

Because Leukine is usually free of side effects, it is rapidly becoming a staple in numerous experimental immune protocols. For example, the Cleveland Clinic has studied combining Leukine with Revlimid, a second-generation type of thalidomide. Revlimid works by suppressing VEGF, an immune-inhibiting hormone commonly released from cancer cells. By doing this, Revlimid actually augments immune activity. When Revlimid was used in combination with Leukine to treat men with relapsed prostate cancer, 70% of the men benefited with some degree of PSA decline.[11]

A BENEFICIAL IMMUNE COCKTAIL

Celebrex, a well-tolerated anti-inflammatory drug approved by the FDA to treat arthritis, has also been shown to inhibit prostate cancer growth.[12] Celebrex inactivates an enzyme called Cox-2 that is overactive in cancer cells. Cox-2 increases the production of prostaglandins, which can also cause immune suppression. Cox-2 also increases VEGF. When blood levels of VEGF are high, tumor cells hide behind this immunosuppressive "cloud" to evade attack from the killer cells. These effects are blocked to some degree when Celebrex inactivates Cox-2. Celebrex is also usually devoid of side effects, making it a good agent to combine with other drugs.

Another such agent, Cytoxan, is a common chemotherapy drug that in very low doses paradoxically stimulates the immune system[13] (as opposed to the standard doses that suppress immunity) by selectively inhibiting the T_{Reg} cells and not allowing the cancer cells to hide behind their suppressive activity.

In our practice, based on the general tolerability of these three drugs, we have been administering Leukine, low-dose Cytoxan and Celebrex in combination to men with relapsed disease during the TIP holiday. We do this in the hope that their immune effects would be additive. So far we have been impressed with the results. Previously rising PSA levels stabilize or decline in about two-thirds of the men we treat.

STARTLING RESULTS WITH IPILIMUMAB

Researchers are finally figuring out how to fully exploit the new realization that cancer has been fooling the immune system by using the T_{Regs} as a shield against immune attack. Medarex, a biopharmaceutical company, has developed a monoclonal antibody called ipilimumab that blocks the activity of CTLA-4, a protein on the surface of the T_{Reg} cells that upregulates T_{Reg} activity. The net effect of blocking CTLA-4 is to reduce T_{Reg} activity and stimulate the immune system. Ipilimumab has been studied in a variety of tumor types. Preliminary studies in small numbers of patients with very advanced prostate cancer have shown some dramatic cancer reversals with sharp PSA declines.

Ipilimumab in combination with TIP lit up the media airwaves when dramatic degrees of cancer regression were observed at the Mayo Clinic in June 2009. The Mayo Clinic press release reads as follows:

Researchers reported that two patients whose prostate cancer had been considered inoperable became cancer free. The supervising physician said, "The approach initiated the death of a majority of cancer cells and caused the tumors to shrink dramatically, allowing surgery. In both cases, the aggressive tumors had grown well beyond the prostate into the abdominal areas. The goal of the study was to see if we could modestly improve upon current treatments for advanced prostate cancer," says Eugene Kwon, MD, the leader of the clinical trial. "The candidates for this study were people who didn't have a lot of other options. However, we were startled to see responses that far exceeded any of our expectations." The patients first received hormone treatment (TIP) resulting in an initial reduction in tumor size. Researchers then introduced a single dose of ipilimumab, an antibody, which stimulates an immune response, resulting in massive death of the tumor cells. Both men experienced consistent drops in their PSA counts over the following weeks until both were deemed eligible for surgery. Then, during surgery, came a greater surprise. "The tumors had shrunk dramatically," says Michael Blute, MD, the urologist, co-investigator and surgeon, who operated on both men. "I had never seen anything like this before. I had a hard time finding the cancer. At one point the pathologist (who was working during surgery) asked if we were sending him samples from the same patient." One patient underwent radiation therapy after surgery; both have resumed their regular lives. Further research is being planned to understand more about the mechanisms of the antibody and how best to use the approach in practice. The researchers, however, note the significance of their findings. "This is one of the holy grails of prostate cancer research," says Dr. Kwon. "We've been looking for this for years."

Although it may be a bit early to conclude that ipilimumab is the miracle cure for prostate cancer, it is one of many new pharmaceutical agents that make the future look very bright. The big pharmaceutical companies obviously recognize their potential. Cougar Biotechnology, the company that developed Abiraterone, was acquired in 2009 by Johnson & Johnson for two billion dollars, and Bristol Myers-Squibb recently purchased Medarex, the maker of ipilimumab for about the same price.

BREAKTHROUGHS ON THE HORIZON CALL
FOR EDUCATED DECISION MAKING

It was the hope of future discoveries that gave me the courage to specialize in medical oncology. When I first started down this path more than twenty years ago, oncology was the bleakest of specialties. Cancer was almost always diagnosed late and the treatments were toxic and ineffective.

My biggest release from the pressures of treating cancer came fifteen years ago when I left general oncology to specialize in prostate cancer. Unlike other common cancers—as I hope Ralph and I have shown— prostate cancer is much less malignant. Improvements in treatment have been slow in coming but they are finally on their way.

At the Active Surveillance Consensus Conference at UCSF in 2007, it was openly bemoaned that the word "cancer" overstates the seriousness of *Low-Risk* disease. However, the pathology experts in attendance shot down proposals for a name change saying, "under the microscope it looks like a cancer, so it's cancer." At that time no one had a rebuttal so the subject was dropped. In retrospect, I wish we had risen to the challenge. When the manufacturers of 7UP faced the problem of distinguishing their product from all the other soft drinks on the market, they came up with a new name, "The Un-Cola," a stroke of marketing genius. My response to the pathology experts is—since they insist that *Low-Risk* disease be called a cancer—let's *un*do the negativity of this word and rename it, "The Un-Cancer." Though *Low-Risk* cancer is indeed cancer, it should in no way be viewed as a death sentence. In fact, it should be regarded as a *chronic* condition.

We have tried to point out throughout this book that the process of selecting treatment can be hobbled by biases and poor information. Some clinics favor a certain type of treatment over all the others because that is "what we do." Academic centers tend to nudge men into experimental research. Insurance companies declare certain new treatments "investigational" and withhold payment because they are not covered.

I see only one conceivable solution to all these challenges. Legislators seem to think that the cost of medicine can be reduced by blocking access to "expensive" specialists. I disagree. Common sense dictates that the least expensive way to do a job is to do it right the first time. Specialists at centers of excellence are in the best position to judge the benefits of new therapies because they have extensive experience with large numbers of patients with the same illness, giving them a much better feel for what is likely to work.

Fortunately, less toxic and more effective new treatments are coming. It is reassuring to know there is no need to rush into treatment without taking time to review all of the options. In this new environment, what was once true only for men with *Low-Risk* cancers like Ralph's can now be said for almost all men with prostate cancer: *Time is on your side.*

THE PATIENT'S VIEW

The message here is heartening. Even for those of us with relapsed prostate cancer, the odds are excellent that with wise choices and proper treatment we will, indeed, die with the disease, not from it.

Mark has spoken often about "the rapidly approaching future." According to Michael Milken's Prostate Cancer Foundation, there are currently more than twenty new prostate cancer therapies in development, and at least sixty new clinical trials each year.

I continue to live with prostate cancer and, yes, sometimes fear of death still riles me up. Yet given the bright future of immune therapy, molecular biology, new drug combinations, research in nanoparticle delivery of prostate cancer medicines, promising new treatment methods now in the pipeline, and the exciting new field of "energy medicine," I am more than ever convinced that of all possible cancers, prostate cancer is the best deal in town.

APPENDIX

AVODART (DUTESTERIDE) AND PROSCAR (FINASTERIDE)

Avodart and Proscar counteract prostate enlargement from benign prostatic hyperplasia (BPH), the enlargement that commonly occurs with aging. These drugs are well tolerated, though under rare circumstances impotence or loss of libido ensues. Proscar and Avodart function by blocking 5-alpha reductase, an enzyme that converts testosterone into dihydrotestosterone (DHT). DHT is the primary hormone inside the prostate gland and is much more potent than testosterone. When the prostate is deprived of DHT, the gland shrinks. By reducing the size of the gland, these medications help reverse the problem of slow urination from prostate enlargement. They are also logical candidates for inhibiting prostate cancer because prostate cancer cells originate directly from the prostate gland and depend on DHT to grow.

PROSCAR FOR PROSTATE CANCER

A study evaluating the effect of Proscar in over 18,000 men was published in the *New England Journal of Medicine* in July of 2003.[1] The stated goal of this study was to determine if Proscar could prevent prostate cancer. However, the study was designed in an era before the prevalence of microscopic *Low-Risk* prostate cancer was appreciated. We now know that almost half the men in the United States over age sixty-five harbor a microscopic amount of low-grade prostate cancer. Therefore a large percentage of the men in the study had preexisting *Low-Risk* prostate cancer at the time of study initiation. Although this research was done to determine if Proscar could prevent prostate cancer, it was really an evaluation of Proscar's effectiveness for treating *existing* prostate cancer.

The study continued for seven years, after which about 10,000 participants had a random six-core prostate biopsy. The men treated with Proscar had 25% fewer cancers of the prostate than the men treated with placebo.

The men on Proscar were also 1% more likely to be diagnosed with *High-Risk* prostate cancer because Proscar improved the accuracy of the PSA monitoring process, making it easier to detect *High-Risk* disease. Unfortunately, in the same issue of the *New England Journal of Medicine*, a famous urologist from Memorial Sloan-Kettering, Peter Scardino, mistakenly assumed that the 1% greater incidence of *High-Risk* disease in the men taking Proscar resulted from the Proscar itself.[2] As implausible as this erroneous conclusion was, the impact of his editorial still lives on, referenced to this day by those with a superficial understanding of the topic. Fortunately, subsequent letters to the editor, as well as a thorough review of the overall issue, demonstrate that this false concern can finally be laid to rest.[3]

So Proscar not only reverses cancer in some men, it also improves the accuracy of the PSA monitoring process by increasing the detection of *High-Risk* cancer.[4]

AVODART

The 5-alpha reductase enzyme exists in three forms. Proscar only blocks the type II form. However, the type I enzyme occurs more commonly in aggressive prostate cancer. Therefore Avodart, a medication that blocks two of the three forms of 5-alpha reductase, may be more effective. There is a study showing that Avodart reduces the likelihood of getting prostate cancer by 22%.[5,6] However, there are no head-to-head studies between Avodart and Proscar to prove one agent is better than the other. For what it's worth, in our practice at Prostate Oncology Specialists we performed a small study in which we checked DHT levels of men on Proscar, then switched them to Avodart and saw a further decline in DHT levels. We found that blood levels of DHT on Avodart were noticeably lower than blood levels on Proscar.

PSA MONITORING

Proscar and Avodart clearly have anti-cancer activity and they both lower PSA. One question that frequently arises is, "Do these agents mask the ability of PSA to signal cancer progression?" The short answer is no. Proscar and Avodart do reset the PSA baseline approximately 50% lower. However, they do not stop PSA from rising in men who have progressive disease. For example, take a man who has a PSA of 6.0 before starting Proscar. The PSA will drop by an average of 50% down to about 3.0. A PSA subsequently rising above 3.0 is a possible indication of cancer progression.[7]

THE PSA STRESS TEST

The lowering effect on PSA can be exploited as a "stress test" in men contemplating going on active surveillance. The vetting process for active surveillance involves various methods to rule out the occult *High-Risk* disease, including a color Doppler ultrasound, endorectal MRI and PCA-3 urine testing. A failure for the typical 50% decline in PSA to occur with the initiation of Proscar or Avodart raises the possibility of unsuspected *High-Risk* disease and may signal the need for a repeat biopsy before active surveillance can safely proceed.[8]

OTHER APPLICATIONS

There are several ways 5-alpha reductase inhibitors can be used. Men who have a family history of prostate cancer can take these agents to reduce their risk. Proscar and Avodart can also be used as inhibitory agents in men with *Low-Risk* disease to prevent progression in men on active surveillance. These drugs can also be used to enhance other more potent testosterone inactivating pharmaceuticals such as Casodex, Eulexin, Lupron, Zoladex and ketoconazole. Only a few studies exist to prove that combining Proscar or Avodart with these other agents improves results, though small studies report positive effects.[9]

There is a strong underlying rationale for believing the addition of Proscar or Avodart is beneficial, as no testosterone inactivating pharmaceutical (Lupron, Casodex, Eligard) eradicates testosterone completely. So an additional nontoxic agent to lower DHT as much as possible seems logical when a maximum anti-cancer effect is needed. The activity of these agents has been demonstrated in other clinical situations: Proscar delays the rise in PSA in men with relapse for a couple of years after surgery.[10] Studies performed at Prostate Oncology Specialists also show that Proscar slows the rate of PSA rise in men on intermittent hormone blockade by doubling the time off or "holiday period."[11]

IS AVODART BETTER THAN PROSCAR?

We are comfortable with both agents. Proscar has the advantage of being less expensive now that it is available in generic form. It also has a twenty-year proven track record of being safe and effective. Avodart may be more potent but there are no head-to-head studies proving superior clinical efficacy.

SIDE EFFECTS

Some side effects can be good. Propecia, another name for Proscar, treats male-pattern baldness. Its effects are modest but usually some improvement can be detected. Another side effect is a beneficial change in urinary flow. Many men taking these agents see a reduction in getting up at night to urinate. On the negative side, a minority of men will note a reduction in sex drive, difficulty getting an erection or breast enlargement. If any of these side effects occur, the treatment should be stopped. The side effects (except for breast enlargement) almost always reverse. A more consistent side effect is a reduction in semen volume, which comes from the fact that these agents reduce the function of the prostate gland.

CONCLUSION

Proscar and Avodart have a good therapeutic ratio. That is, they have a meaningful therapeutic effect with minimal side effects. They are user friendly in that they don't interact with other medications and can be taken any time of the day with or without food. Proscar is available as a generic (finasteride) and is very affordable. Given all these advantages, some doctors are considering their use in men who are yet to be diagnosed with prostate cancer in order to prevent the disease. Although they may prove valuable in this capacity, we have found these agents to be more useful in the therapeutic sense, to treat prostate cancer after it has been diagnosed.

NOTES

CHAPTER 2

1. Ian Thompson, *The influence of finasteride on the development of prostate cancer*. New England Journal of Medicine, July 2003.
2. Hermann Brenner, *Long-term survival rates of patients with prostate cancer in the prostate-specific antigen era: Population-based estimate for the year 2000 by period analysis*. Journal of Clinical Oncology, January 2005.
3. Joseph Cappelleri, *Analysis of single items on the self-esteem and relationship questionnaire in men treated with sildenafil citrate for erectile dysfunction: results of two double-blind, placebo-controlled trials*. British Journal of Urology, April 2008.
4. Brian Quaranta, *Comparing radical prostatectomy and brachytherapy for localized prostate cancer*. Oncology, September 2004.
5. Edan Shapiro, *Long-term outcomes in younger men following permanent prostate brachytherapy*. Journal of Urology, April 2009.
6. Catherine Buron, *Brachytherapy versus prostatectomy in localized prostate cancer: Results of a French multicenter prospective medico-economic study*. International Journal of Radiation Oncology Biology Physics, March 2007.

CHAPTER 4

1. Peter Scardino, *Early detection of prostate cancer*. Human Pathology, March 1992.
2. Hermann Brenner, *Long-term survival rates of patients with prostate cancer in the prostate-specific antigen era: Population-based estimate for the year 2000 by period analysis*. Journal of Clinical Oncology, January 2005.
3. Anthony D'Amico, *Predicting prostate-specific antigen outcome preoperatively in the prostate-specific antigen era*. Journal of Urology, December 2001.
4. Grace Lu-Yao, *Effect of age and surgical approach on complications and short-term mortality after radical prostatectomy—a population-based study*. Urology, August 1999.
5. John Mulhall, *Defining and reporting erectile function outcomes after radical prostatectomy: Challenges and misconceptions*. Journal of Urology, February 2009.

6. Harin Padma-Nathan, *Postoperative nightly administration of sildenafil citrate significantly improves the return of normal spontaneous erectile function after bilateral nerve-sparing radical prostatectomy*. Journal of Urology, Abstract 1402, 2003.
7. Marc Savoie, *A prospective study measuring penile length in men treated with radical prostatectomy for prostate cancer*. Journal of Urology, April 2003.
8. Sean Elliott, *Incidence of urethral stricture after primary treatment for prostate cancer: Data from CaPSURE*. Journal of Urology, August 2007.
9. Patrick Walsh, *Patient-reported urinary continence and sexual function after anatomic radical prostatectomy*. Urology, January 2000.
10. Paul Lange, *Views from the "other side": Personal reflections about prostate cancer from two urological oncologists*: Prostate Cancer: Principles and Practice, April 2006.
11. Philipp Dahm, *A longitudinal assessment of bowel related symptoms and fecal incontinence following radical perineal prostatectomy*. Journal of Urology, June 2003.
12. James Eastham, *Variations among individual surgeons in the rate of positive surgical margins in radical prostatectomy specimens*. Journal of Urology, December 2003.
13. Anna Bill-Axelson, *Radical prostatectomy versus watchful waiting in localized prostate cancer group-4 randomized trial*. Journal of the National Cancer Institute, August 2008.
14. Amy Krambeck, *Radical prostatectomy for prostatic adenocarcinoma: a matched comparison of open retropubic and robot-assisted techniques*. British Journal of Urology International, February 2009.
15. F. R. Schroeck, *Satisfaction and regret after open retropubic and robot-assisted laparoscopic radical prostatectomy*. European Urology, October 2008.

CHAPTER 6

1. Judd Moul, *Early versus delayed hormonal therapy for prostate-specific antigen only recurrence of prostate cancer after radical prostatectomy*. Journal of Urology, March 2004.
2. Laurence Klotz, *Active surveillance for prostate cancer: For whom?* Journal of Clinical Oncology, November 2005.
3. Rhonda Walsh, *Prostate cancer screening may have an unintended effect on survival and mortality—the camel's nose effect*. Journal of Urology, April 2007.
4. Stephen Boorjian, *Mayo Clinic validation of the D'Amico risk group classification for predicting survival following radical prostatectomy*. Journal of Urology, April 2008.

5. Ballentine Carter, *Expectant management of nonpalpable prostate cancer with curative intent: An update of the Johns Hopkins experience.* Journal of Urology, December 2007.

6. Manish Patel, *An analysis of men with clinically localized prostate cancer who deferred definitive therapy.* Journal of Urology, April 2004.

7. Barbara Ercole, *Outcomes following active surveillance of men with localized prostate cancer diagnosed in the prostate-specific antigen era.* Journal of Urology, October 2008.

8. Mark Soloway, *Active surveillance: A reasonable management alternative for patients with prostate cancer: The Miami experience.* British Journal of Urology International, 2007.

9. Roderick van den Bergh, *Outcomes of men with screen-detected prostate cancer eligible for active surveillance who were managed expectantly.* European Urology, January 2009.

10. Anthony Zeitman, *Active surveillance: A safe, low-cost prognostic test for prostate cancer.* British Journal of Urology International, 2008.

CHAPTER 8

1. Gerald Andriole, *Mortality results from a randomized prostate-cancer screening trial.* New England Journal of Medicine, March 2009.

2. Fritz Schroder, *Screening and prostate-cancer mortality in a randomized European study.* New England Journal of Medicine, March 2009.

3. Unnur Valdimarsdottir, *Completed suicides among newly diagnosed prostate cancer patients.* Genitourinary Cancer Symposium, Abstract 104, February 2008.

4. Fang Fang, *Cardiovascular events among newly diagnosed prostate cancer patients.* Genitourinary Cancer Symposium Abstract 12, February 2008.

5. Larissa Rodriguez, *Risks and complications of transrectal ultrasound guided prostate needle biopsy: A prospective study and review of the literature.* Journal of Urology, December 1998.

6. Altug Tuncel, *The impact of transrectal prostate needle biopsy on sexuality in men and their female partners.* Urology, July 2008.

7. Amnon Zisman, *The impact of prostate biopsy on patient well-being: a prospective study of pain, anxiety and erectile dysfunction.* Journal of Urology, February 2001.

8. Ralf Kurek, *Quantitative PSA RT-PCR for preoperative staging of prostate cancer.* The Prostate, June 2003.

9. Michael Oefelein, *Clinical and molecular follow up after radical retropubic prostatectomy.* Journal of Urology, August 1999.

10. Ian Thompson, *Operating characteristics of prostate-specific antigen in men*

with an initial PSA level of 3.0 ng/mL or lower. Journal of the American Medical Association, December 2005.

11. Robert Allan, *Correlation of minute (0.5 mm or less) focus of prostate adenocarcinoma on needle biopsy with radical prostatectomy specimen: Role of prostate-specific antigen density.* Journal of Urology, August 2003.

12. Stacy Loeb, *PSA doubling time versus PSA velocity to predict High-Risk prostate cancer: Data from the Baltimore longitudinal study of aging.* European Urology, July 2008.

13. Chris Griffin, *Trial of empiric antibiotics prior to recommending biopsy for PSA elevation helps stratify prostate cancer risk.* Journal of Urology, Abstract 1790, May 2009.

14. Hiroyuki Nakanishi, *PCA3 molecular urine assay correlates with prostate cancer tumor volume: Implications for selecting candidates for active surveillance.* Journal of Urology, May 2008.

15. Ian Thompson, *Chemoprevention of Prostate Cancer.* Journal of Urology, August 2009.

CHAPTER 10

1. Judd Moul, *Early versus delayed hormonal therapy for prostate-specific antigen only recurrence of prostate cancer after radical prostatectomy.* Journal of Urology, March 2004.

2. Mark Scholz, *Prostate cancer-specific survival and clinical progression-free survival in men with prostate cancer treated intermittently with testosterone inactivating pharmaceuticals.* Urology, September 2007.

3. Martin Gleave, *Randomized comparative study of 3 versus 8-month neoadjuvant hormonal therapy before radical prostatectomy: Biochemical and pathological effects.* Journal of Urology, August 2001.

4. Paddy Niblock, *Rising prostate-specific antigen values during neoadjuvant androgen deprivation therapy: The importance of monitoring.* International Journal of Radiation Oncology Biology Physics, May 2006.

5. Mark Scholz, Re: *Recovery of spontaneous erectile function after nerve-sparing radical prostatectomy with and without early intracavernous injections of alprostadil: Results of a prospective randomized trial.* Journal of Urology, Letter, June 1999.

6. Nancy Keating, *Diabetes and cardiovascular disease during androgen deprivation therapy for prostate cancer.* Journal of Clinical Oncology, September 2006.

7. Christopher Saigal, *Androgen deprivation therapy increased cardiovascular morbidity in men with prostate cancer.* Cancer, July 2007.

8. Anthony D'Amico, *Influence of androgen suppression therapy for prostate*

cancer on frequency and timing of fatal myocardial infarctions. Journal of Clinical Oncology, June 2007.

9. Michel Bolla, *Duration of androgen suppression in the treatment of prostate cancer.* New England Journal of Medicine, June 2009.

10. Fritz Schroder, *Early versus delayed endocrine treatment of T2-T3 pN1-3 MO prostate cancer without local treatment of the primary tumor: Final results of European organization for the research and treatment of cancer protocol 30846 after 13 years of follow-up.* European Urology, September 2008.

11. Jason Efstathiou, *Cardiovascular mortality after androgen deprivation therapy for locally advanced prostate cancer: RTOG 85-31.* Journal of Clinical Oncology, January 2009.

12. Urs Studer, *Immediate or deferred androgen deprivation for patients with prostate cancer not suitable for local treatment with curative intent: European organization for research and treatment of cancer (EORTC) trial 30891.* Journal of Clinical Oncology, April 2006.

13. Payam Hakimian, *Metabolic and cardiovascular effects of androgen deprivation therapy.* British Journal of Urology International, August 2008.

14. Jennifer Yannucci, *The effect of androgen deprivation therapy on fasting serum lipid and glucose parameters.* Journal of Urology, August 2006.

15. Stephen Strum, *Anemia associated with androgen deprivation in patients with prostate cancer receiving combined hormone blockade.* British Journal of Urology, June 1997.

CHAPTER 12

1. James Eastham, *Predicting an optimal outcome after radical prostatectomy: The Trifecta Nomogram.* Journal of Urology, June 2008.

2. Peter Grimm, *10-year biochemical (prostate-specific antigen) control of prostate cancer with ^{125}I brachytherapy.* International Journal of Radiation Oncology Biology Physics, April 2002.

3. Stephen Freedland, *Prostate cancer update: 2004.* Reviews in Urology, October 2005.

4. Steven Leibel, *Prostate Cancer: Three-dimensional conformal and intensity-modulated radiation therapy.* PPO Updates, Principles & Practice of Oncology, 2000.

5. Shabbir Alibhai, *Examining the location and cause of death within 30 days of radical prostatectomy.* British Journal of Urology International, March 2005.

6. Leslie Yonemoto, *Combined proton and photon conformal radiation therapy for locally advanced carcinoma of the prostate: preliminary results of a phase I/II study.* International Journal of Radiation Oncology Biology Physics, March 1997.

7. David Hernandez, *Contemporary evaluation of the D'Amico risk classification of prostate cancer.* Urology, November 2007.

8. John Sylvester, *15-year biochemical relapse free survival in clinical stage T1-T3 prostate cancer following combined external beam radiotherapy and brachytherapy; Seattle experience.* International Journal of Radiation Oncology Biology Physics, January 2007.

CHAPTER 14

1. John Kurhanewicz, *Prostate cancer: Prediction of extracapsular extension with endorectal MRI and three-dimensional proton MR spectrographic imaging.* Radiology, November 1999.

2. Penelope Wood, *The role of combined MRI and MRSI in treating prostate cancer.* PCRI Insights, August 2000.

3. Hedvig Hricak, *Validity of prostate-specific antigen as a tumor marker in watchful waiting prostate cancer patients: Correlation with findings at serial endorectal magnetic resonance imaging and spectroscopic imaging.* British Journal of Urology, January 2007.

4. Martin Umbehr, *Combined magnetic resonance imaging and magnetic resonance spectroscopy imaging in the diagnosis of prostate cancer: A systematic review and meta-analysis.* European Urology, March 2009.

5. Alexander Kirkham, *How good is MRI at detecting and characterizing cancer within the prostate?* European Urology, June 2006.

6. Anthony D'Amico, *Role of percent positive biopsies and endorectal coil MRI in predicting prognosis in intermediate-risk prostate cancer patients.* Cancer Journal from Scientific American, 1996.

7. Duke Bahn, *Color doppler and tissue harmonic ultrasound in the early detection and staging of prostate cancer.* PCRI Insights, November 2002.

8. Jeong Cho, *Peripheral hypoechoic lesions of the prostate: Evaluation with color and power doppler ultrasound.* European Urology, April 2000.

9. Ferdinand Frauscher, *Comparison of contrast enhanced color doppler targeted biopsy with conventional systematic biopsy: Impact on prostate cancer detection.* Journal of Urology, April 2002.

10. Michael Mitterberger, *Comparison of contrast enhanced color dopper targeted biopsy to conventional systematic biopsy: Impact on Gleason score.* Journal of Urology, August 2007.

11. Robert Bree, *The role of color doppler and staging biopsies in prostate cancer detection.* Urology, March 1997.

12. Duke Bahn, *Focal prostate cryoablation: Initial results show cancer control and potency preservation.* Journal of Endourology, September 2006.

13. Erica Lambert, *Focal cryosurgery: Encouraging health outcomes for unifocal prostate cancer.* Urology, June 2007.

14. Manfred Wirth, *Antiandrogens in the treatment of prostate cancer.* European Urology, February 2007.

CHAPTER 16

1. Stephen Boorjian, *Mayo Clinic validation of the D'Amico risk group classification for predicting survival following radical prostatectomy.* Journal of Urology, April 2008.
2. Michel Bolla, *Long-term results with immediate androgen suppression and external irradiation in patients with locally advanced prostate cancer (an EORTC study): a phase II randomized trial.* The Lancet, July 2002.
3. Anthony D'Amico, *6-month androgen suppression plus radiation therapy vs radiation therapy alone for patients with clinically localized prostate cancer.* Journal of the American Medical Association, August 2004.
4. Miljenko Pilepich, *Androgen deprivation with radiation therapy compared with radiation therapy alone for locally advanced prostatic carcinoma: A randomized comparative trial of the radiation therapy oncology group.* Urology, April 1995.
5. John Davis, *Quality of life after treatment for localized prostate cancer: Differences based on treatment modality.* Journal of Urology, September 2001.
6. John Wei, *Comprehensive comparison of health-related quality of life after contemporary therapies for localized prostate cancer.* Journal of Clinical Oncology, January 2002.
7. James Talcott, *Time course and predictor of symptoms after primary prostate cancer therapy.* Journal of Clinical Oncology, November 2003.
8. David Miller, *Long-term outcomes among localized prostate cancer survivors: Health-related quality-of-life changes after radical prostatectomy, external radiation, and brachytherapy.* Journal of Clinical Oncology, April 2005.
9. Stephen Frank, *An assessment of quality of life following radical prostatectomy, high dose external beam radiation therapy and brachytherapy iodine implantation as monotherapies for localized prostate cancer.* Journal of Urology, June 2007.
10. Martin Sanda, *Quality of life and satisfaction with outcome among prostate-cancer survivors.* New England Journal of Medicine, March 2008.
11. Mark Scholz, Re: *Recovery of spontaneous erectile function after nerve-sparing radical prostatectomy with and without early intracavernous injections of alprostadil: Results of a prospective randomized trial.* Journal of Urology, Letter, June 1999.
12. Roanne Segal, *Resistance exercise in men receiving androgen deprivation therapy for prostate cancer.* Journal of Clinical Oncology, May 2003.
13. M. Hammar, *Acupuncture treatment of vasomotor symptoms in men with prostate cancer: A pilot study.* Journal of Urology, March 1999.

14. Fergus Coakley, *Urinary continence after radical retropubic prostatectomy: Relationship with membranous urethral length on preoperative endorectal magnetic resonance imaging.* Journal of Urology, September 2002.

15. Peter Scardino, *Continuing refinements in radical prostatectomy: More evidence that technique matters.* Journal of Urology, February 2005.

16. Paolo Gontero, *New insights into the pathogenesis of penile shortening after radical prostatectomy and the role of postoperative sexual function.* Journal of Urology, August 2007.

17. Colin Begg, *Variations in morbidity after radical prostatectomy.* New England Journal of Medicine, April 2002.

18. Pierre Karakiewicz, *Thirty-day mortality rates and cumulative survival after radical retropubic prostatectomy.* Urology, December 1998.

19. John Mulhall, *Defining and reporting erectile function outcomes after radical prostatectomy: Challenges and misconceptions.* Journal of Urology, February 2009.

20. Harin Padma-Nathan, *Postoperative nightly administration of sildenafil citrate significantly improves the return of normal spontaneous erectile function after bilateral nerve-sparing radical prostatectomy.* Journal of Urology, Abstract 1402, 2003.

21. Amy Marcus, *Prostate surgery preserves potency but HMO's are putting up barriers.* Wall Street Journal, June 2002.

CHAPTER 18

1. Michio Kushi, *The Cancer Prevention Diet: Michio Kushi's Macrobiotic Blueprint for the Prevention and Relief of Disease.* New York: St. Martin's Griffin, 1994.

2. Verne Varona, *Nature's Cancer Fighting Foods: Prevent and Reverse the Most Common Forms of Cancer Using the Proven Power of Great Food and Easy Recipes.* Paramus, NJ: Reward Books, 2001.

3. Dean Ornish, *Intensive lifestyle changes may affect the progression of prostate cancer.* Journal of Urology, September 2005.

4. Carmen Rodriguez, *Diabetes and risk of prostate cancer in a prospective cohort of U.S. men.* American Journal of Epidemiology, January 2005.

5. Ann Hsing, *Prostate cancer risk and serum levels of insulin and leptin: A population-based study.* Journal of the National Cancer Institute, May 2001.

6. Livia Augustin, *Glycemic index, glycemic load and risk of prostate cancer.* International Journal of Cancer, 2004.

7. Steven Lehrer, *Serum insulin level, disease stage, prostate-specific antigen (PSA) and Gleason score in prostate cancer.* British Journal of Cancer, October 2002.

8. Samantha Bowker, *Increased cancer related mortality for patients with type 2 diabetes who use sulfonyureas or insulin.* Diabetes Care, February 2006.
9. Josie Evans, *Metformin reduces risk of cancer in diabetic patients.* British Medical Journal, June 2005.
10. Ben Sahra, *The antidiabetic drug metformin exerts an antitumoral effect in vitro and in vivo through a decrease in cyclin D1 level.* Oncogene, January 2008.
11. Stephen Freedland, *Body mass index as a predictor of prostate cancer: development versus detection on biopsy.* Urology, July 2005.
12. Lillian Hsieh, *Association of energy intake with prostate cancer in a long-term aging study: Baltimore longitudinal study of aging (United States).* Urology, February 2003.
13. Stephen Freedland, *Obesity and risk of biochemical progression following radical prostatectomy at a tertiary care referral center.* Journal of Urology, September 2005.
14. Christopher Amling, *Pathologic variables and recurrence rates as related to obesity and race in men with prostate cancer undergoing radical prostatectomy.* Journal of Clinical Oncology, February 2004.

CHAPTER 20

1. David Crawford, *Epidemiology of prostate cancer.* Urology, December 2003.
2. Lillian Hsieh, *Association of energy intake with prostate cancer in a long-term aging study: Baltimore longitudinal study of aging (United States).* Urology, February 2003.
3. Stephen Freedland, *Obesity and risk of biochemical progression following radical prostatectomy at a tertiary care referral center.* Journal of Urology, September 2005.
4. Marion Lee, *Soy and isoflavone consumption in relation to prostate cancer risk in China.* Cancer Epidemiology, Biomarkers & Prevention, July 2003.
5. Tomoko Sonoda, *A case-control study of diet and prostate cancer in Japan: Possible protective effect of traditional Japanese diet.* Cancer Science, March 2004.
6. Bjarne Jacobsen, *Does high soy milk intake reduce prostate cancer incidence? The Adventist Health Study (United States).* Cancer Causes Control, December 1998.
7. Lon White, *Brain aging and midlife tofu consumption.* Journal of the American College of Nutrition, April 2000.
8. Amanda Cross, *A prospective study of meat and meat mutagens and prostate cancer risk.* Cancer Research, December 2005.
9. R. James Barnard, *A low-fat diet and/or strenuous exercise alters the IGF axis in vivo and reduces prostate tumor cell growth in vitro.* The Prostate, August 2003.

10. Michael Pollak, *Insulin-like growth factors and neoplasia.* Nature Reviews Cancer, July 2004.

11. June Chen, *Insulin-like growth factor-I (IGF-I) and IGF binding protein-3 as predictors of advanced-stage prostate cancer.* Journal of the National Cancer Institute, July 2002.

12. Paul Terry, *Fatty fish consumption and risk of prostate cancer.* The Lancet, June 2001.

13. Katarina Augustsson, *A prospective study of intake of fish and marine fatty acids and prostate cancer.* Cancer Epidemiology, Biomarkers & Prevention, January 2003.

14. Carmen Rodriguez, *Calcium, dairy products, and risk of prostate cancer in a prospective cohort of United States men.* Cancer Epidemiology, Biomarkers & Prevention, July 2003.

15. Li-Qiang Qin, *Milk consumption is a risk factor for prostate cancer: Meta-analysis of case-control studies.* Nutrition and Cancer, January 2004.

16. Camilla Hoppe, *Animal protein intake, serum insulin-like growth factor I, and growth in healthy 2.5-y-old Danish children.* American Journal of Clinical Nutrition, August 2004.

17. Jian Xu, *Serum levels of phytanic acid are associated with prostate cancer risk.* The Prostate, May 2005.

18. Edward Giovannucci, *A prospective study of tomato products, lycopene, and prostate cancer risk.* Journal of the National Cancer Institute, March 2002.

19. Mahyar Etminan, *The role of tomato products and lycopene in the prevention of prostate cancer: A meta-analysis of observational studies.* Cancer Epidemiology, Biomarkers & Prevention, March 2004.

20. A. Duffield-Lillico, *Selenium supplementation baseline plasma selenium status and incidence of prostate cancer: An analysis of the complete treatment period of the Nutritional Prevention of Cancer Trial.* British Journal of Urology, May 2003.

21. Scott Lippman, *Effect of selenium and vitamin E on risk of prostate cancer and other cancers.* Journal of the American Medical Association, January 2009.

22. Olli Heinonen, *Prostate cancer and supplementation with alpha-tocopherol and beta-carotene: Incidence and mortality in a controlled trial.* Journal of the National Cancer Institute, March 1998.

23. Edgar Miller, *Meta-analysis: High-dosage vitamin E supplementation may increase all-cause mortality.* Annals of Internal Medicine, January 2005.

24. B. Greg Brown, *Simvastatin and niacin, antioxidant vitamins, or the combination for the prevention of coronary disease.* New England Journal of Medicine, November 2001.

25. Michael Joseph, *Cruciferous vegetables, genetic polymorphisms in glutathione*

s-transferase m1 and t1, and prostate cancer risk. Nutrition and Cancer, January 2004.

26. Coleman Gross, *Treatment of early recurrent prostate cancer with 1,25-dihydroxyvitamin D3 (Calcitriol).* Journal of Urology, June 1998.

27. Laufey Steingrimsdottir, *Relationship between serum parathyroid hormone levels, vitamin D sufficiency, and calcium intake.* Journal of the American Medical Association, November 2005.

28. June Chan, *Dairy products, calcium and vitamin D and risk of prostate cancer.* Epidemiologic Reviews, January 2001.

29. Edward Giovannucci, *Calcium and fructose intake in relation to risk of prostate cancer.* Cancer Research, February 1998.

30. Karla Lawson, *Multivitamin use and the risk of prostate cancer in the national institutes of health-AARP diet and health study.* Journal of the National Cancer Institute, May 2007.

31. M. Leitzmann, *Zinc supplement use and risk of prostate cancer.* Journal of the National Cancer Institute, July 2003.

CHAPTER 22

1. Michael Oefelein, *Skeletal fractures negatively correlate with overall survival in men with prostate cancer.* Journal of Urology, September 2002.

2. Hakan Melhus, *Excess dietary intake of vitamin A is associated with reduced bone mineral density and increased risk of hip fracture.* Annals of Internal Medicine, November 1998.

3. Harry Daniell, *Osteoporosis after orchiectomy for prostate cancer.* Journal of Urology, February 1997.

4. Eric Small, *Osteoporosis in men treated with androgen deprivation therapy for prostate cancer.* Journal of Urology, May 2002.

5. Matthew Smith, *Low bone mineral density in hormone-naïve men with prostate cancer.* Cancer, June 2001.

6. Jonathan Myers, *Exercise capacity and mortality among men referred for exercise testing.* New England Journal of Medicine, March 2002.

7. Roanne Segal, *Resistance exercise in men receiving androgen deprivation therapy for prostate cancer.* Journal of Clinical Oncology, May 2003.

CHAPTER 24

1. Judd Moul, *Early versus delayed hormonal therapy for prostate-specific antigen only recurrence of prostate cancer after radical prostatectomy.* Journal of Urology, March 2004.

2. Mark Scholz, *Intermittent use of testosterone inactivating pharmaceuticals using finasteride prolongs the time-off period.* Journal of Urology, May 2006.

3. Fernando Calais da Silva, *Intermittent androgen deprivation for locally advanced and metastatic prostate cancer: Results from a randomized phase 3 study of the south European uroncological group.* European Urology, June 2009.

4. Jean de Leval, *Intermittent versus continuous total androgen blockade with advanced hormone-naïve prostate cancer: Results of a prospective randomized trial.* Clinical Prostate Cancer, December 2002.

5. Ulf Tunn, *The current status of intermittent androgen deprivation (IAD) therapy for prostate cancer: Putting IAD under the spotlight.* British Journal of Urology International, January 2007.

6. Per-Anders Abrahamsson, *Potential benefits of intermittent androgen suppression therapy in the treatment of prostate cancer: A systematic review of the literature.* European Urology, January 2010.

7. Michael Milano, *A prospective pilot study of curative-intent stereotactic body radiation therapy in patients with 5 or fewer oligometastatic lesions.* Cancer, December 2007.

8. Mack Roach, *Phase III trial comparing whole-pelvic versus prostate-only radiotherapy and neoadjuvant versus adjuvant combined androgen suppression: Radiation therapy oncology group 9413.* Journal of Clinical Oncology, May 2003.

9. Colleen Lawton, *RTOG GU radiation oncology specialists reach consensus on pelvic lymph node volumes for high-risk prostate cancer.* International Journal of Radiation Oncology Biology Physics, June 2009.

10. Brian Rini, *Clinical and immunological characteristics of patients with serologic progression of prostate cancer achieving long-term disease control with granulocyte-macrophage colony-stimulating factor.* Journal of Urology, June 2006.

11. R. Dreicer, *Phase I/II study of lenalidomide (Revlimid®) and GM-CSF (Leukine®) in hormone refractory prostate cancer (HRPC).* Journal of Clinical Oncology, Abstract, June 2007.

12. Raj Pruthi, *Phase II trial of Celecoxib in prostate-specific antigen recurrent prostate cancer after definitive radiation therapy or radical prostatectomy.* Clinical Cancer Research, April 2006.

13. K. Bass, *Immunopotentiation with low-dose cyclophosphamide in the active specific immunotherapy of cancer.* Cancer Immunology, Immunotherapy, September 1998.

APPENDIX

1. Ian Thompson, *The influence of finasteride on the development of prostate cancer.* New England Journal of Medicine, July 2003.

2. Peter Scardino, *The prevention of prostate cancer—The dilemma continues.* New England Journal of Medicine, July 2003.

3. Claus Roehrborn, *Prevention of prostate cancer with finasteride.* New England Journal of Medicine, October 2003.
4. Ian Thompson, *Effect of finasteride on the sensitivity of PSA for detecting prostate cancer.* Journal of the National Cancer Institute, August 2006.
5. Gerald Andriole, *Effect of dutasteride on the detection of prostate cancer in men with benign prostatic hyperplasia.* Urology, 2004.
6. Gerald Andriole, *Further analysis from the REDUCE prostate cancer risk reduction trial.* Journal of Urology, April 2009.
7. Gerald Andriole, *Treatment with finasteride preserves usefulness of prostate-specific antigen in the detection of prostate cancer: Results of a randomized, double-blind, placebo-controlled clinical trial.* Urology, August 1998.
8. Steven Kaplan, *PSA response to finasteride challenge in men with a serum PSA greater than 4 ng/ml and previous negative prostate biopsy: Preliminary study.* Urology, 2002.
9. Oliver Sartor, *Activity of dutasteride plus ketoconazole in castration-refractory prostate cancer after progression on ketoconazole alone.* Clinical Genitourinary Cancer, October 2009.
10. Gerald Andriole, *Treatment with finasteride following radical prostatectomy for prostate cancer,* Urology, March 1995.
11. Mark Scholz, *Intermittent use of testosterone inactivating pharmaceuticals using finasteride prolongs the time-off period.* Journal of Urology, May 2006.

ACRONYMS

ASTRO: American Society for Therapeutic Radiation and Oncology.

BPH (BENIGN PROSTATIC HYPERPLASIA): Benign swelling of the prostate gland that occurs with aging. BPH also can cause elevation of PSA and problems with urination.

DHT: See DIHYDROTESTOSTERONE in glossary.

DNA (DEOXYRIBONUCLEIC ACID): The basic biologically active chemical that defines the physical development and growth of nearly all living organisms; a complex protein that is the carrier of genetic information.

DRE: DIGITAL RECTAL EXAMINATION

Dx: Standard abbreviation for diagnosis.

ECTM: See EMOTIONAL-CHEMICAL TEXT MESSAGES in glossary.

IGF-1 (INSULIN-LIKE GROWTH FACTOR-1): Hormone released by the liver in response to growth hormone. IGF-1 is the substance that stimulates the tissues to grow.

IMRT (INTENSITY MODULATED RADIATION THERAPY): An approach to radiation therapy allowing the treatment team to specify the tumor target dose and the amount of radiation allowable to the nearby tissues and employing sophisticated computer planning.

MRI (MAGNETIC RESONANCE IMAGING): A scanning technology that creates images of the soft tissues and internal organs by using a powerful magnetic field. Sometimes a contrast agent will be injected into a vein, usually gadolinium, to create brighter images.

PCA-3: Urine test used to detect prostrate cancer. A high score is suggestive of larger amounts of higher grade cancer.

PET (POSITRON EMISSION TOMOGRAPHY): Scanning technique that uses injected radioactive glucose to localize cancerous tumors within the body.

PSA (PROSTATE-SPECIFIC ANTIGEN): PSA is a glycoprotein. It is normally present in the blood stream, produced by the epithelial cells of the prostate for the ejaculate, allowing sperm to swim freely and it dissolves the cervical mucous cap so that sperm may enter the uterus. PSA is also secreted by prostate cancer cells. An elevated PSA level in the blood indicates an abnormal condition of the prostate gland, either benign or malignant, or an infection. An elevated PSA has been known to result from recent ejaculation, infection or BPH.

RAD: A unit of absorbed radiation dose.

TGF-b (TRANSFORMING GROWTH FACTOR BETA): A bone-derived growth factor that stimulates the prostate cancer cell and osteoblast, among many other functions.

TIP (TESTOSTERONE INACTIVATING PHARMACEUTICALS): Medicines that block the action of the male hormone testosterone and cause prostate cancer regression.

TRUS (TRANSRECTAL ULTRASOUND): A method that uses echoes of ultrasound waves (far beyond the hearing range) to image the prostate by inserting an ultrasound probe into the rectum; commonly used to visualize and guide prostate biopsy procedures.

TURP (TRANSURETHRAL RESECTION OF THE PROSTATE): A surgical procedure to remove tissue obstructing the urethra. The technique involves the insertion of an instrument called a resectoscope into the penile urethra, and is intended to relieve obstruction of urine flow due to enlargement of the prostate.

VEGF (VASCULAR ENDOTHELIAL GROWTH FACTOR): A substance known to stimulate blood vessel growth or angiogenesis and hence stimulate tumor growth.

GLOSSARY

ABLATION: Relating to the removal or destruction of tissue or a system; androgen ablation refers to blocking the effects of androgens by surgical or chemical means.

ACTIVE SURVEILLANCE: Active observation and regular monitoring of a patient without actual treatment.

ADENOCARCINOMA: A form of cancer that develops from a malignant abnormality in the cells lining a glandular organ such as the prostate; almost all prostate cancers are adenocarcinomas.

ADJUVANT THERAPY: An additional treatment used to increase the effectiveness of the primary therapy; radiation therapy is often used as an adjuvant treatment after a radical prostatectomy if the surgical margins are positive.

AEROBIC: In biochemistry, chemical reactions that require oxygen.

ALLOPATHIC MEDICINE: Allopath from Greek *állos*, "other," "different" and *páthos*, "suffering." Licensed MDs practice allopathic medicine. Also called traditional or conventional medicine, as opposed to homeopathic or naturopathic medicine.

ANAEROBIC: An organism or a cell that can live in the absence of atmospheric oxygen.

ANDROGEN: A hormone responsible for male characteristics and the development and function of male sexual organs (e.g., testosterone) produced mainly by the testicles. Androgens have far-reaching effects on blood formation, muscle and bone mass, cognitive function, emotion, skin and hair.

ANDROGEN DEPRIVATION THERAPY: Also called hormone therapy, or testosterone inactivating pharmaceuticals (TIP). A prostate cancer treatment that eliminates or blocks chemical castration, antiandrogens, 5-alpha reductase inhibitors, estrogenic compounds, agents that interfere with adrenal androgen production, agents that decrease sensitivity of the androgen receptor.

ANGIOGENESIS: The growth of new blood vessels. Angiogenesis is a normal biologic process that occurs in both healthy and disease states, as well as in wound healing. Without angiogenesis, a tumor cannot grow beyond a certain size.

ANTIOXIDANT: A substance that inhibits oxidation or reactions promoted by oxygen or peroxides. Antioxidant nutrients protect human cells from damage caused by free radicals (highly reactive oxygen compounds).

APOPTOSIS: Programmed cell death due to an alteration in a critical substance or chemical necessary for cell viability; the lack of male hormones causes apoptosis in cancer cells that are androgen dependent.

ATHEROSCLEROSIS: Commonly known as hardening of the arteries. Arterial blood vessels are involved, the arterial walls thicken, there is a buildup of fatty materials such as cholesterol, and there is a chronic inflammatory response in the walls of arteries.

BENIGN PROSTATIC HYPERPLASIA OR HYPERTROPHY (BPH): Noncancerous condition of the prostate resulting in the growth of both glandular and stromal (supporting connective) tumorous tissue that can enlarge the prostate and obstruct urination.

BRACHYTHERAPY: A form of radiation therapy in which radioactive seeds or pellets that emit radiation are implanted within the prostate in order to destroy the cancer.

CALCIFICATION: Impregnation with calcium or calcium salts.

CAPSULAR PENETRATION: Tumor extending through the wall of the prostate, outside the gland.

CAPSULE: The fibrous tissue that acts as an outer lining of the prostate.

CAT SCAN (CT OR COMPUTERIZED AXIAL TOMOGRAPHY): A method of combining images from multiple x-rays under the control of a computer to produce cross-sectional or three-dimensional pictures of the internal organs.

CLINICAL STAGE: Prostate cancer stage as determined by digital rectal examination.

COLLATERAL DAMAGE: A side effect, or a reaction to a medication or treatment.

COMBINED HORMONAL THERAPY: The use of more than one variety of hormone therapy, especially the use of LHRH analogs (e.g., Lupron, Zoladex) to block the production of testosterone by the testes, plus antiandrogens (e.g., Casodex [bicalutamide], Eulexin [flutamide], Anandron [nilutamide], or Androcur [cyproterone]) to compete with DHT and with testosterone for cell androgen receptors, thereby depriving cancer cells of DHT and testosterone needed for growth; also referred to as CHB, TIP, MAB, ADT and TAB.

CONFORMAL THERAPY: An older radiation technique designed to focus external radiation on the prostate and protect surrounding organs and areas that do not require treatment.

CORE: A tissue sample removed during biopsy.

DENDRITIC CELLS: Cells that process antigens (proteins) and present them to immune lymphocytes called T cells playing a major role in the initiation of the immune response against tumors and other types of abnormal cells.

DIFFERENTIATION: The use of the differences between prostate cancer cells when seen under the microscope as a method to grade the severity of the disease. Well-differentiated cells are easily recognized as normal cells, whereas poorly differentiated cells are abnormal, cancerous and difficult to recognize as belonging to any particular type of cell group.

DIHYDROTESTOSTERONE (DHT OR 5-ALPHA DIHYDROTESTOSTERONE): A male hormone more potent than testosterone that is converted from testosterone within the prostate by an enzyme called 5-alpha reductase (see Appendix).

DOUBLING TIME: The time that it takes a value (like PSA) to double.

EMOTIONAL-CHEMICAL TEXT MESSAGES (ECTM): An on/off switching mechanism that determines immune system functioning. According to the theory articulated by Deepak Chopra, MD, that every cell in the body is "eavesdropping on our thoughts and feelings," we are constantly "text messaging" to the immune system, and those messages either activate its healing function or place it on alert for fight-or-flight, in which instance the healing function is switched off.

EPIDIDYMIS: Tightly coiled, thin-walled tube that conducts sperm from the testes to the vas deferens and provides for the storage, transmission and maturation of sperm.

EXTERNAL BEAM RADIATION THERAPY (EBRT): A form of radiation therapy in which the radiation is delivered by a machine directed at the area to be radiated, as opposed to radiation given within the target tissue such as brachytherapy; external beam radiation treatment can include conventional photons or use protons, neutrons or electrons. This treatment may be given conventionally or with 3D conformal techniques; see also IMRT.

EXTRA-CAPSULAR EXTENSION: Cancer extending beyond the prostate capsule.

FOCAL THERAPY: A more localized treatment directed at the cancerous foci within the gland, rather than removing or destroying the entire prostate.

FOSSA: The niche in the pelvis that is created when the prostate gland is surgically removed.

FREE RADICAL: An atom or group of atoms that has at least one unpaired electron and is therefore unstable and highly reactive. In animal tissues, free radicals can damage cells and are believed to accelerate the progression of cancer, cardiovascular disease and age-related diseases.

GLEASON GRADE: A widely used method for classifying prostate cancer tissue for the degree of loss of the normal glandular architecture (size, shape and differentiation of glands); a grade from 1–5 is assigned successively to each of the two most predominant tissue patterns present in the examined tissue sample and the two grades are added together to produce the Gleason score; high numbers indicate poor differentiation and therefore more aggressive cancer.

GLEASON SCORE: Two Gleason grade numbers are added together to produce the Gleason score. The first number indicates the Gleason grade of the cancer cells found most commonly within the sample and the second number is the second most commonly found grade. For example, a Gleason score of 4 + 3 = 7 means that Gleason grade 4 is the most commonly found type of cell and Gleason grade 3 is the second most commonly found, producing a total Gleason score of 7. Gleason score is grouped into low-grade (2–6), intermediate-grade (7) and high-grade (8–10).

HORMONE THERAPY: The use of hormones, hormone analogs and certain surgical techniques to treat disease either on their own or in combination with other hormones.

IMMUNOTHERAPY: Treatment of disease by inducing, enhancing or suppressing an immune system response.

INTERMITTENT ANDROGEN DEPRIVATION: Discontinuing testosterone lowering therapy to allow the patient to recover from symptoms and side effects of low testosterone.

KILLER CELLS: White blood cells that attack tumor cells and normal cells that have been invaded by viruses.

LESION: A localized pathological change in a bodily organ or tissue. Tumors are considered lesions.

LOCAL TREATMENT: Treatment that includes generally accepted procedures necessary to ultimately produce recovery of the patient. For prostate cancer this usually includes radical prostatectomy, radiation therapy and cryosurgery.

LYMPH NODES: The small glands that occur throughout the body and filter the clear fluid known as lymph or lymphatic fluid; lymph nodes filter out bacteria and other toxins as well as cancer cells.

MARGIN: Normally used to mean the "surgical margin," which is the boundary or outer edge of the tissue removed during surgery. If the surgical margin shows no sign of cancer (negative margins), then the prognosis is better.

METASTASIS: A secondary tumor formed as a result of a cancer cell or cells from the primary tumor site (e.g., the prostate) traveling through the body to a different location in the body.

MONOTHERAPY: A treatment that uses one major drug or one major modality of treatment, such as using only an LHRH.

MUTATION: A change in the genetic material (DNA) inside the cell.

NEOVASCULARITY: New blood vessel growth, particularly as relates to providing a blood supply to a tumor.

NERVE SPARING: A type of prostatectomy in which the surgeon attempts to save the nerves that affect sexual function.

NEUROVASCULAR BUNDLES: Two bundles of nerves on the surface of the prostate that control erection.

ONCOLOGY: The branch of medicine dealing with tumors (cancer). The term originates from the Greek, derived from *onkos*, meaning bulk, mass or tumor, and the suffix *-logy*, meaning "study of" or "to talk about."

PALPABLE: Capable of being felt during a physical examination by an experienced physician. In the case of prostate cancer, this normally refers to some form of abnormality of the prostate that can be felt during a digital rectal examination.

PATHOLOGIST: A physician who specializes in the examination of tissues and blood samples to decide what diseases or abnormalities are present.

PERINEUM: The area of the body between the scrotum and the anus; a perineal procedure uses this area as the point of entry into the body.

PERINEURAL INVASION: Prostate cancer invading the nerve sheath surrounding the nerves that enter the prostate.

PITUITARY GLAND: A small endocrine gland at the base of the brain that supplies hormones that control many body processes, including the production of testosterone by the testes.

PLACEBO: A nonactive treatment frequently used as a basis for comparison with pharmaceuticals in research studies. Approximately 25% of all placebos produce results equivalent to those obtained by actual treatment or drugs.

POSITIVE MARGIN: The pathologic finding of cancer cells on the outer edge of the tissue removed.

PROCTITIS: Inflammation of the rectum; in prostate cancer therapy this may be associated with radiation therapy.

PROSTATE: From Greek *prostates*, meaning "one who stands before," "protector" or "guardian." It is an exocrine gland of the male reproductive system. About the size of a walnut when healthy, it surrounds the urethra and sits immediately below the bladder. Its function is to make, store and excrete a milky white, alkaline fluid that helps to neutralize the acidity of the vagina and allows the sperm to live for approximately seventy-two hours, providing better motility and better protection of the genetic material (DNA). The prostate also has smooth muscles to help expel semen ejaculate. It requires the male hormones testosterone and dihydrotestosterone to function properly.

PROSTATITIS: A bacterial infection or inflammation of the prostate gland. An ailment ranging from acute, requiring immediate medical attention, to chronic, lasting more than three months, to asymptomatic.

PSA DENSITY: The amount of PSA per unit volume of the prostate gland (see chapter 8).

PSA DOUBLING TIME: The time it takes for the PSA value to double. A significant factor in prostate cancer staging.

PSA VELOCITY: The calculation of the rate of increase in PSA levels in succeeding PSA tests; before diagnosis, a PSA velocity of 0.4 ng/ml/year (or higher) may be an indication of the presence of cancer.

RANDOMIZED: The process of assigning patients to different forms of treatment in a research study in a random manner.

RELAPSE: The return of signs and symptoms of cancer following a period of improvement.

REMISSION: The real or apparent disappearance of some or all of the signs and symptoms of cancer; the period (temporary or permanent) during which a disease remains under control without progressing; even complete remission does not necessarily indicate cure.

SEED, SEEDING: Permanent brachytherapy: brachytherapy from the Greek *brachy*, meaning "short-distance." The permanent implantation of radioactive seeds or pellets (also called capsules), which emit low to high energy radiation in order to kill surrounding tissue, for example, the prostate, including prostate cancer cells. Also known as "seed implantation."

SEMINAL VESICLES: Glandular structures located above and behind the prostate that secrete and store seminal fluid; the seminal vesicles connect with the ejaculatory ducts and contain nutrients for the sperm that improve their viability and mobility.

SEMINAL VESICLE INVASION OR INVOLVEMENT: Prostate cancer cells that are found outside the prostate in the seminal vesicle(s) or have migrated to the seminal vesicle(s) from a prostate tumor.

SURGICAL MARGINS: The outer edge or boundary of the tissue removed during surgery.

SYNERGISTIC: Having the ability to assist or add to the activity of another substance, such as a drug.

T CELL: An immune system cell that orchestrates an immune response to infected or malignant cells, sometimes by direct contact with the abnormal cells. T-cells are lymphocytes that develop in the thymus and bone marrow and circulate in the blood and lymphatic system (see dendritic cell).

TESTOSTERONE: The male hormone or androgen that comprises most of the androgens in a man's body, chiefly produced by the testicles but also derived from adrenal androgen precursors such as DHEA and androstenedione. It is highly important to a man's sexual interest or libido and his ability to achieve erection. Testosterone plays a key role in virtually every tissue in the human body (e.g., brain, bone, blood formation, skin, nails and muscle).

TESTOSTERONE INACTIVATING PHARMACEUTICALS (TIP): Also known as androgen deprivation therapy (ADT) or hormone therapy.

TOMOTHERAPY: A form of intensity-modulated radiation therapy that uses a CT scanner to direct the radiation beam.

VACUUM ERECTION DEVICE (VED): A device that creates an erection with a vacuum. It is usually a hard, plastic device placed over the penis, a vacuum is then created by a pump, bringing blood into the penis.

VAS DEFERENS: From the Latin *ductus deferens* "carrying-away vessel," (plural: vasa deferentia). The vasa are two ducts through which sperm travel from the testes to the prostate prior to ejaculation. It is the vas deferens that is cut in the male form of contraception known as a vasectomy.

ANNOTATED BIBLIOGRAPHY

Men newly diagnosed with prostate cancer, those at risk for the disease and, most particularly, their wives and partners, may want additional information that is not part of this book's mission. Titles listed here present both traditional and nontraditional ways of managing and treating prostate cancer. Certain of these titles—such as those by Groopman, Lipton, and Weil—are just plain good reading.

Symbols: books particularly recommended by the patient (**P**), and by the doctor (**D**)

BARBARA and RALPH ALTEROWITZ, *Intimacy with Impotence: The Couple's Guide to Better Sex after Prostate Disease*, First DaCapo Life Long Books, Cambridge, MA, 2004. The essential resource for couples trying to reestablish intimacy and sex in the face of impotence. *The Lovin' Ain't Over* (Westbury, NY, Health Education Literary Publisher), by the same authors, is also helpful. **P**

GREG ANDERSON, *Cancer: 50 Essential Things to Do*, Plume Book Penguin-Putnam, New York, 1999. Anderson founded the Cancer Recovery Foundation of America. He was diagnosed with cancer and given thirty days to live. He interviews 16,000 cancer survivors to find the things to which they attributed getting well and recommends forming "strategies and action points" about how to "take control" of your cancer. He also recommends reframing cancer as a challenge to make you a better person—a turning point to give you a brighter future. Love what your cancer can do for you if you are willing to take up the challenge. Author of six other books including: *Healing Wisdom, The Cancer Conqueror* and *The 22 (Non-Negotiable) Laws of Wellness*. **P**

JAMES BALCH, MD, and PHYLLIS BALCH, CNC, *Prescriptions for Nutritional Healing*, 4th ed., Penguin Group, Avery, New York, 2006. Dr. Balch is a fellow of the American College of Surgeons and the author of five books on health and nutrition. Phyllis Balch is a nutritional counselor and advocate of natural therapies. This is a basic book about selecting and using vitamins, minerals and herbs as dietary supplements. **P**

DAVID BOSTWICK, DAVID CRAWFORD, CELESTIA S. HIGANO, and MACK ROACH, *American Cancer Society's Complete Guide to Prostate Cancer*,

American Cancer Society, 2005. This book offers a safe adherence to the established way of doing things. It is written by sixty-two prominent people in the field, all speaking about their specialty. A humanizing touch is the insertion throughout of photographs of men who are quoted about their experiences. **P**

GLEN BUBLEY, MD, and WINIFRED CONKLING, *What Your Doctor May Not Tell You about Prostate Cancer*, Warner Books, New York, 2005. The title suggests secrets revealed and a better way of doing things, but this turns out not to be the case. For men with advanced cancer, however, the book is informative, particularly in chapters about experimental treatments and clinical trials that were already under way several years ago.

COLIN CAMPBELL, PhD, and THOMAS CAMPBELL II, *The China Study*, BenBella Books, Dallas, TX. Links diets high in animal-based protein (including casein in cow's milk) with disease and cancer. A study comparing diet, lifestyle and disease characteristics in sixty-five counties in rural China in the 1970s and 1980s conducted jointly by Cornell University, Oxford University and the Chinese Academy of Preventive Medicine. The authors recommend that people eat a whole food, plant-based diet and avoid consuming pork, beef, game, poultry, fish, eggs and milk as a means to minimize and/or reverse the development of chronic disease. **P, D**

BARRIE CASSILETH, PhD, *The Alternative Medicine Handbook: The Complete Reference Guide to Alternative and Complementary Therapies*, W.W. Norton, New York, 1999. This excellent book is out of print but worth hunting down. The author founded the Integrative Medicine Service at the Memorial Sloan-Kettering Cancer Center, where she holds the Laurence S. Rockefeller Chair in Integrative Medicine. She also founded the Society for Integrative Oncology. **P**

VICTOR CHENEY, *Castration: The Advantages and Disadvantages*, 1st Books Library, 1993. A surprisingly interesting and informative book on the history of castration. The book contains a wealth of information about the subject, the politics and the unusual (to a lay person) aspects of the procedure. The author, who devoted twenty-five years to the study of castration treatment, underwent castration himself for prostate cancer and is without regrets.

HOLLY CLEGG and GERALD P. MITELLO, MD, *Eating Well through Cancer*, Favorite Recipes Press, Nashville, TN, 2001, 2006. Holly Glegg, author of healthy eating books such as *Trim and Terrific*, has teamed with Gerald Mitello, a medical oncologist of twenty years practice and research who recognizes the importance of diet and nutrition before and after treatment. Extensive information and great recipes! **P**

MICHAEL DORSO, *Seeds of Hope: A Physician's Personal Triumph over Prostate Cancer*, Acorn Publishing, Battle Creek, MI, 2000. Written by an emergency room physician with the aggressive type of the disease who chose to treat his cancer with a combination of hormones, beam radiation and radiation seed therapy, Dorso writes well about the decision-making process, expounding on the benefits and negative aspects of his decisions as well as the impact of the cancer on his wife and himself. A useful and heartening book for men considering radiation seed therapy.

JEROME GROOPMAN, MD, *How Doctors Think*, Houghton Mifflin, Boston, MA, 2007. This is an enlightening examination and clarification of the thinking styles of doctors, a translation between doc-think and patient-think. The book demystifies medicine, giving patients the tools they need to improve their dealings with health care professionals. The author challenges readers to examine their own assumptions about the medical world. **P**

RICHARD HARDY, *Prostate Cancer: Treatment and Recovery*, Prometheus Books, Amherst, NY, 1996. This book vividly examines the psychological effects of impotence—vulnerabilities, indignities, depression—both on the author and on his wife. Men contemplating treatments that potentially cause impotence who are unclear about all its ramifications will find the book very informative.

BRADLEY HENNENFENT, MD, *Surviving Prostate Cancer without Surgery*, Roseville Books, Roseville, IL, 2005. This is an easy-to-read book that deals graphically and honestly with the shortcomings of surgery.

AARON KATZ, MD, *Dr. Katz's Guide to Prostate Health*, Freedom Press, Topanga, CA, 2006. A sound and helpful overview of both traditional and alternative treatments. Includes thoughtful descriptions of state-of-the-art techniques and research.

SIMON KELLY and ENRIDA KELLY, *Healing Cancer: The Top 12 Non-Toxic Cancer Treatments to Help You Beat Cancer*, The London Press, London, UK, 2005. If you consult only one book on this field, it might well be this one. It provides accurate and responsible guidance on the latest and most important nontoxic cancer treatments, based on the knowledge and experience of seven of the world's leading professionals in this field. Detailed information about each nontoxic therapy is discussed, including cost and availability. There are good data on leading conventional cancer clinics and how to utilize the therapies they offer. The authors also introduce a remarkable human resource: Etienne Callebout. **P**

MICHAEL KORDA, *Man to Man: Surviving Prostate Cancer*, Random House, New York, 1996. This book is an extremely well written and accurate description of the author's odyssey through prostate surgery. This is one of the first books to lay bare the risks of post-op problems with incontinence and impotence, even when surgery is performed by the best surgeon in the country. Graphically portrays what it's really like to undergo a radical prostatectomy. **D**

MICHIO KUSHI and ALEX JACK, *The Cancer Prevention Diet*, St. Martin's Griffin, New York, 1993. Little directly relating to prostate cancer (about twelve pages) but this book is a sound and comprehensive "blueprint" for fighting cancer with a macrobiotic diet. The first author is the acknowledged leader of the international macrobiotic community and natural foods movement. **P**

LARRY LACHMAN, PHD, and RIC MASTEN, *Parallel Journeys: A Spirited Approach to Coping & Living with Cancer*, Sunink Presentations, Carmel, CA. 2003. Two cancer survivors, one a clinical psychologist, the other a poet/philosopher, tell their stories and pool their wisdom and experience. An informal yet authoritative overview and specific approach to living through prostate cancer.

PAUL LANGE, MD, and CHRISTINE ADAMEC, *Prostate Cancer for Dummies*, Wiley, New York, 2003. First-rate general overview of the traditional approach to prostate cancer treatment written by a urologist who himself had prostate surgery. The information is presented in easy-to-access and simple form. Good on coping with stress. Rich with information to make an informed decision. **P, D**

BRUCE LIPTON, PHD, *The Biology of Belief: Unleashing the Power of Consciousness, Matter, & Miracles*, Hay House, Carlsbad, CA, 2008. Also *Spontaneous Evolution: A Positive Future and a Way to Get There from Here*, Hay House, Carlsbad, CA, 2009. Lipton, a cell biologist and epigeneticist, is one of those rare people who is best described as "an adventurer in ideas." You needn't have cancer to benefit from his creative thinking. **P**

SHELDON MARKS, MD, *Prostate Cancer: A Family Guide to Diagnosis, Treatment, and Survival*, 3rd ed., Perseus, New York, 2003. Originally published in 1995, written by a urologist, this book focuses largely on the standard treatment provided by urologists. A useful book, thanks to an easy-to-use question-and-answer format and a good index.

EMIL I. MONDOA, MD, and MINDY KITEI, *Sugars That Heal*, Ballantine Books, New York, 2001. This book offers a revolutionary new health plan based on the evolving science of glyconutrients—foods that contain saccharides. For our bodies to function properly we need small amounts of eight essential sugars. When all eight are included in our diet we can increase our ability to fight disease, activate the immune system, lower cholesterol, increase lean muscle, decrease body fat, ease allergy symptoms and ward off infections and disease. **P**

MARK MOYAD, MD, *Dr. Moyad's No BS Health Advice: A Step-by-Step Guide to What Works and What's Worthless*, Ann Arbor Media Group, 2008. Dr. Moyad provides an easy-to-read overview of some of the common health issues, especially as related to dietary supplements. **P, D**

JOHN P. MULHALL, MD, *Sexual Function in the Prostate Cancer Patient*, Humana Press, New York, 2009. Written by an impressive lineup of experts and edited by perhaps the preeminent expert in erectile dysfunction for men after treatment for prostate cancer. **D**

JOHN P. MULHALL, MD, *Saving Your Sex Life: A Guide for Men with Prostate Cancer*, Hilton Publishing, Chicago, IL, 2008. This book guides sexually active men with prostate cancer through the pitfalls and side effects of treatments and how to avoid them. It is an outstanding guide for men with prostate-related sexual dysfunction and their wives or partners. **P**

CHARLES "SNUFFY" MYERS, MD, *Beating Prostate Cancer: Hormonal Therapy and Diet*, Rivanna Health Publications, 2007. One of the few books that presents TIP as a feasible method of first-line therapy, written by one of the best translators of medical jargon into lay language. Dr. Myers, himself a prostate cancer survivor and one of the foremost experts of the field, writes a most readable introduction to these important topics. **P, D**

DEAN ORNISH, MD, *The Spectrum*, Random House, New York, 2007. An empowering book from the man who pioneered research into the way diet and lifestyle changes can reverse heart disease. Ornish is now doing further groundbreaking research on changes in prostate gene expression in men undergoing intensive nutritional and lifestyle intervention. **P**

PATRICK QUILLIN, PhD, RD, CNS, *Beating Cancer with Nutrition*, Nutrition Times Press, Carlsbad, CA, 2009, revised. A major resource for cancer nutrition issues, including an appendix with a list of nutritionally oriented doctors throughout the U.S. For ten years, Quillin was Director of Nutrition for the Cancer Treatment Centers of America. **P**

ERNEST E. ROSENBAUM, MD, FACP, and ISADORA ROSENBAUM, MA, *Everyone's Guide to Cancer Supportive Care*, Andrews McMeel, Kansas City, MO, 2005. I found the Rosenbaums' book to be useful, refreshing and full of good ideas from biofeedback as a tool for cancer management to visualization (an excellent presentation of Carl Simonton's work), to nine steps for practicing "the Art of Forgiveness." A truly user-friendly and rewarding book. **P**

STEVEN ROSENBLATT, MD, PhD, and CAMERON STAUTH, *The Starch Blocker Diet*, Harper Collins, New York, 2003. Useful nutrition and diet book, with recipes, that explains how to eat the foods we love without hunger and lose weight by neutralizing calories safely and instantly and stabilizing blood sugars. **P**

PETER SCARDINO and JUDITH KELMAN, *Dr. Peter Scardino's Prostate Book: The Complete Guide to Overcoming Prostate Cancer, Prostatitis and BPH*, Avery, New York, 2005. Written by the chief of urology at Memorial Sloan-Kettering, the most prestigious cancer hospital in the world, this book presents the quintessential surgeon's viewpoint.

DAVID SERVAN-SCHREIBER, MD, PhD, *Anticancer: A New Way of Life*, Viking Penguin, New York, 2009. A neuroscientist and brain cancer survivor, the author has created a "blueprint" for living that focuses on supplementing conventional medical treatment with integrative and complementary dietary measures. The glossy color middle section on food groupings, what to eat, what to avoid and what actually inhibits cancer cell growth is brilliant. This book is a formidable contribution to the field. Servan-Schreiber's website: www.anticancerbook.com. **P**

EUGEN SHIPPEN MD, and WILLIAM FRYER, *The Testosterone Syndrome: The Critical Factor for Energy, Health & Sexuality — Reversing the Male Menopause*. M. Evans, New York, 1998. All you will ever want to know about testosterone — and then some.

BERNIE S. SIEGEL, MD, *Peace, Love & Healing*, Harper & Row, New York, 1989. Follow-up to his previous bestseller, *Love, Medicine & Miracles*, Harper & Row, 1986. This is a surgeon's inspiring view of mind–body communication and the path to self-healing. Heartwarming accounts of exceptional patients show the critical role we can play in our own recovery. **P**

CARL SIMONTON, MD, STEPHANIE MATTHEWS-SIMONTON, and JAMES CREIGHTON, *Getting Well Again: A Step-by-Step, Self-Help Guide to Overcoming Cancer for Patients and Their Families*, Bantam Books, New York, 1978. Simonton is arguably the godfather of "visualizing recovery." A lot to be said in favor of his work. **P**

STEPHEN STRUM, MD, and DIANA POGLIANO, *A Primer on Prostate Cancer: The Empowered Patient's Guide*, Life Extension Media, Hollywood, FL, 2002. This book provides an encyclopedia of prostate cancer data, with in-depth information about all treatment approaches. **D**

Fuller Torrey, MD, *Surviving Prostate Cancer: What You Need to Know to Make Informed Decisions*, Yale University Press Health & Wellness, New Haven, CT, 2006. Well-organized, comprehensive and informative. An extensive guide to the challenges facing every man diagnosed with this disease.

Verne Varona, *Nature's Cancer Fighting Foods*, Reward Books, Paramus, NJ, 2001. Macrobiotics made accessible, set in a form of "macrobiotics lite" for the benefit of western readers. Solid explanations, recommendations and dietary programs. A useful book in an area gaining more and more attention. Also recently released: *Macrobiotics for Dummies*, Wiley, Hoboken, NJ, 2009, by the same author. **P, D**

Barbara Wainrib and Sandra Haber, *Men, Women, and Prostate Cancer*. New Harbinger, Oakland, CA, 2000. Revised version of a 1996 book, *A Guide for Women and the Men They Love*. Written by two psychologists for the wives of men with prostate cancer. Strong on emotional issues. There is a good chapter on how to respond to your man's impotence. **P**

Patrick Walsh, MD, and Janet F. Worthington, *Dr. Patrick Walsh's Guide to Surviving Prostate Cancer*, Wellness Central, New York, 2007. An encyclopedic review of how to treat newly diagnosed prostate cancer from the quintessential urologist's perspective. The book reflects the surgical predisposition of the senior author, who is famous for inventing nerve-sparing prostate surgery. **P**

Andrew Weil, MD, *Spontaneous Healing: How to Discover and Enhance Your Body's Natural Ability to Maintain and Heal Itself*, Alfred A. Knopf, New York, 1995. Weil is a member of the admirable company that includes Carl Simonton, Bernie Siegel, Larry Dossey and Bruce Lipton. In clear, concise language, he explains how the human healing system operates, "its interactions with the mind, its biological organization, its systems of self-diagnosis, self-repair, and regeneration." A basic book for the burgeoning field of mind–body medicine. As is frequently the case with such seminal works, Weil provides an appendix: "Finding Practitioners, Supplies and Information." **P**

Chuck Wheeler and Martha Wheeler, *Affirming the Darkness: An Extended Conversation about Living with Prostate Cancer*, Memoirs Unlimited, Beverly, MA, 1996. This husband and wife of fifty years kept separate diaries from the time of Wheeler's diagnosis until his death eight years later. Their book takes a clear-eyed look at surgery, penile prosthesis, orchiectomy (castration), metastasis, pain control and dying of the disease. The strength of this couple's love for each other makes reading this book a powerful and often moving experience.

PROSTATE ONCOLOGISTS: A PRELIMINARY LIST

As we have pointed out, prostate cancer is the only common cancer managed by surgeons. One of the most frequent reasons men consult me as a medical oncologist is that I am thought to be free of bias, at least as far as deciding between radiation and surgery is concerned. Unfortunately, there is no register of medical oncologists whose primary concern is prostate cancer. With extensive contributions from Jim O'Hara and Jan Manarite from the Prostate Cancer Research Institute Helpline, we have compiled a preliminary list that is by no means all-inclusive, since there is no special licensing or training that would enable us to track down every prostate oncologist in this country or abroad. Most of the medical oncologists included here are at universities. The majority appeared on our radar because at some point they published journal articles on the subject of prostate cancer. However, we are unable to provide information regarding their competency or skills. We can only confirm that they are medical oncologists and that they have taken a particular interest in prostate cancer.

—MARK SCHOLZ

Prostate Oncologists

Name	Phone	State	City	Institution
Agus, David	310-272-7640	CA	Los Angeles	USC Westside Prostate Cancer Center
Bander, Neil H.	212-746-5460	NY	New York	Weill Cornell Medical Center
Beer, Tomasz	503-494-8534	OR	Portland	OHSU Cancer Care Center
Brouns, Matthew	360-944-9889	OR	Portland	Oregon Health Sciences University
Brufsky, Adam	412-647-2811	PA	Pittsburgh	University of Pittsburgh School of Medicine
Buchholtz, Michael S.	631-470-4958	NY	Greenlawn	
Carducci, Michael	410-614-3977	MD	Baltimore	Johns Hopkins Hospital
Cesarman-Maus, Gabriela	011-525-533-1855	Mexico	Mexico City	Institute of Internal Medicine
Chatta, Gurkamal	412-692-4724	PA	Pittsburgh	U. of Pittsburgh, Hillman Cancer Center
Chi, Kim	604-985-4818	BC	Vancouver, Canada	Vancouver Prostate Center
Cusan, Leonello	418-654-2704	PQ	Quebec	Laval University
Dawson, Nancy	202-444-4922	DC	Washington	Lombardi Comprehensive Cancer Center
De Bono, Johann	44-207-352-8171	UK	London	Institute of Cancer Research, Royal Marsden Hospital
Diamond, Pierre	418-654-2704	PQ	Quebec, Canada	Laval University
DiPaola, Robert	732-235-7469	NJ	New Brunswick	Cancer Center of NJ, Robert Wood Johnson Medical School
Dorff, Tanya	323-865-3905	CA	Los Angeles	USC Keck School of Medicine
Eisenberger, Mario	410-955-7955	MD	Baltimore	Johns Hopkins Hospital
Ferrari, Anna	212-731-5389	NY	New York	NYU Cancer Institute
Fizazi, Karim	33 1 42 11 45 53	France	Paris	Institut Gustav-Roussy
Figg, William Douglas	301-402-3622	MD	Bethesda	NIH, Med. Branch Developmental Therapeutics Dept.
Galen, William	503-228-6509	OR	Portland	

Name	State	City	Institution	Phone
Garnick, Marc	MA	Boston	Beth Israel Deaconess Medical Center	617-374-9047
Gomez, Jose-Luis	PQ	Quebec, Canada	Laval University	418-654-2704
Gross, Mitchell	CA	Los Angeles	USC Westside Prostate Cancer Center	310-272-7600
Higano, Celestia	WA	Seattle	University of Washington, Seattle Cancer Care Alliance	208-288-6542
Hudes, Gary	PA	Philadelphia	Fox Chase Cancer Center	215-728-2754
Hussain, Maha Hadi	MI	Ann Arbor	U-M Comprehensive Cancer Center	734-936-8906
Kantoff, Philip	MA	Boston	Dana-Farber/Harvard Cancer Center	617-632-1914
Kelly, William Kevin	CT	New Haven	Yale Cancer Center	203-785-4095
Koletsky, Alan	FL	Boca Raton	Center for Hematology-Oncology	561-955-6400
Kosty, Michael	CA	La Jolla	Scripps Clinic, Green Cancer Center	858-455-9100
Lam, Richard	CA	Marina del Rey	Prostate Oncology Specialists	310-827-7707
Leibowitz, Robert	CA	Los Angeles	Compassionate Oncology Med. Group	310-229-3555
Lindberg, Peter	NM	Los Alamos	Los Alamos Medical Center	505-662-3450
Logothetis, Christopher	TX	Houston	Dept of GU Medical Oncology, MD Anderson Hospital	713-792-2121
Morris, Michael	NY	New York	Memorial Sloan Kettering	646-497-9068
Myers, Charles "Snuffy"	VA	Earlysville	American Institute for Diseases of the Prostate	434-964-0212
Oh, William K.	NY	New York	Mount Sinai Medical Center	800-637-4624
Oliver, Tim	UK	London	The Royal London Hospital	44-0171-377-7000
Petrylak, Daniel	NY	New York	Columbia Presbyterian University Medical Center	212-305-5098
Picus, Joel	MO	St. Louis	Washington University Medical School	314-362-5740
Pienta, Kenneth	MI	Ann Arbor	University of Michigan Comprehensive Cancer Center	734-647-3421
Pinski, Jacek	CA	Los Angeles	USC Keck School of Medicine	323-865-3929
Quesada, Jorge R.	TX	Houston	UT Physicians	823-325-7100

Name	Phone	State	City	Institution
Quinn, David	800-USC-CARE	CA	Los Angeles	USC Keck School of Medicine
Raghavan, Derek	216-445-6888	OH	Cleveland	Taussig Cancer Center, Cleveland Clinic
Redfern, Charles	858-637-7888	CA	San Diego	Oncology Associates of San Diego
Rettig, Matthew B.	310-206-2434	CA	Los Angeles	UCLA Jonsson Comprehensive Cancer Center
Ryan, Charles	415-353-7171	CA	San Francisco	UCSF Helen Diller Cancer Center
Sartor, Oliver	504-988-7869	LA	New Orleans	Tulane Medical School
Scher, Howard I.	646-497-9068	NY	New York	Memorial Sloan Kettering
Scholz, Mark C.	310-827-7707	CA	Marina del Rey	Prostate Oncology Specialists
Shevrin, Daniel	847-570-2112	IL	Evanston	Evanston Kellogg Cancer Center
Small, Eric J.	415-353-7171	CA	San Francisco	UCSF Urologic Oncology Program
Smith, Matthew	617-724-5257	MA	Boston	Harvard/Mass General Hospital
Stadler, Walter	773-702-6149	IL	Chicago	University of Chicago Medical Center
Sternberg, Cora	39-06-5870-4356	Italy	Rome	San Camillo Forlanini Hospital
Strum, Stephen	541-201-0219	OR	Ashland	
Tisman, Glenn	562-789-8822	CA	Whittier	
Trump, Donald	716-845-2300	NY	Buffalo	Roswell Park Cancer Institute
Tucker, Steven	65-68836968 310-5943301	Singapore		Pacific Cancer Center
Ueno, Winston Mizuo	703-823-5322	VA	Alexandria	Fairfax Northern Virginia Hematology Oncology Alexandria
Vogelzang, Nicholas J.	702-952-3400	NV	Las Vegas	Comprehensive Cancer Center
Yu, Evan	206-288-6542	WA	Seattle	U. of Washington, Seattle Cancer Care Center

WEB SITES

American Cancer Society

www.cancer.org

Has chapters in most major cities and provides information on diagnoses and conventional treatment options. Also sponsors Man-to-Man, an online support group for men with prostate cancer.

Cancer Recovery Foundation of America

www.cancerrecovery.org

Gives information on integrated cancer care. Compares conventional, complementary and alternative treatments. Experts actually answer the phone!

CancerCare

www.cancercare.org

A nonprofit organization that provides free professional support services including financial assistance.

Diet and Nutrition Web Sites

American Dietetic Association

www.eatright.org

Offers general nutrition information for the public and helps identify registered dieticians in your area.

American Institute for Cancer Research

www.aicr.org

Consolidates global research information on prevention, diet and exercise.

Jeanne Blum, MT, OMT

www.womanhealthyself.com

Click on the "For Men" button for answers to questions about cancer symptoms, diet and potency.

Kushi Institute

www.kushiinstitute.org

The leading educational organization for macrobiotics.

University of California Prostate Cancer Nutrition Monograph
http://cancer.ucsf.edu/crc/nutrition_prostate.pdf
A well-researched, user-friendly tool for learning about the role of diet in prostate cancer and how to make dietary changes.

Geffen Visions International, Inc.

www.geffenvisions.com
A healthcare education, research and consulting company, specializing in integrative medicine and oncology, offering a leading-edge, multidimensional approach to medicine and wellness, based on Dr. Jeremy Geffen's pioneering program, The Seven Levels of Healing.

Malecare

www.malecare.com
Live online support groups of experienced patients, and doctors who write weekly updates on treatments and their side effects. The organization facilitates cancer support groups for gay men throughout the country. Information on the Web site is available in Spanish, French, Italian and Russian.

National Center for Complementary and Alternative Medicine

www.nccam.nih.gov
Half the population of the U.S. uses alternative and complementary medical practices that are listed here, along with reliable, well-researched information about those practices and therapies.

National Cancer Institute

www.cancer.gov
The NCI's Cancer Information Service (CIS) has trained staff who answer questions, send out relevant literature, refer you to resources in your area, and provide state-of-the-art information concerning treatment protocols and ongoing clinical trials.

Prostate Cancer Canada Network

www.cpcn.org
A national association of more than 100 cancer support groups. Good on diagnosis, treatment, support groups, recommended reading.

Prostate Cancer Foundation (PCF)

www.PCF.org
Provides comprehensive information (including new drugs, clinical trials, latest research, support groups) and resources.

Prostate Care Today

www.prostatecaretoday.com

Valuable resource for African-American men and their families. How to access all basic information from free screening to ethnicity-determined disease.

Prostate Cancer Research Institute (PCRI)

www.prostate-cancer.org

Provides state-of-the-art information and a free subscription to "Insights," a prostate cancer newsletter.

The Prostate Forum

www.prostateforum.com

Since 1996 Dr. "Snuffy" Myers' Prostate Forum Newsletter has been delivering in-depth prostate cancer information to patients, their loved ones and health professionals in easy-to-understand language and with meticulous attention to hard science.

The Prostate Net

www.prostate-online.org

Provides information and support to help patients decide which courses of action offer the best chance for cure and retaining quality of life, increase awareness of prostate cancer risks, simplify the treatment decision-making process through education, and provide access to the tools needed by patients' families and friends to support their decisions.

Us TOO International, Inc.

www.ustoo.org

This worldwide, grassroots organization, started in 1990 by prostate cancer survivors, provides resources to educate and support prostate cancer patients and their caregivers, partners, families and friends. The site lists over 300 support groups nationwide.

Women Against Prostate Cancer (WAPC)

www.womenagainstprostatecancer.org

A national organization working to provide support for the millions of women affected by prostate cancer, and their families. WAPC advocates prostate cancer education, screenings, legislation, and treatment options.

OTHER PUBLICATIONS BY SCHOLZ AND BLUM

M. Scholz & R. Blum, "Who's Really at Risk for What? A Perspective on Prostate Cancer in Relation to Heart Attacks, Osteoporosis, Colon Cancer, Sarcopenia, Lung Cancer, Melanoma," *PCRI Insights*, 7: 2005.

M. Scholz & R. Blum, "Managing the Side Effects of Testosterone Inactivating Pharmaceuticals" (TIP). *PAACT*, 20: 2005.

M. Scholz & R. Blum, "Can Diet Really Control Prostate Cancer?" *PCRI Insights*, 9: 2006.

BOOKS BY RALPH H. BLUM

The Book of Runes, New York, St. Martin's Press, 25th Anniversary Edition, 2008.

The Relationship Runes, with Bronwyn Jones, St. Martin's Press, New York, 2003.

The Healing Runes, with Susan Loughan, St. Martin's Press, New York, 1995.

The Book of Rune Cards, Oracle Books, St. Martin's Press, New York, 1989.

Beyond Earth: Man's Contact with UFOs, with Judy Blum, Bantam Books, New York, 1975.

Old Glory & the RealTime Freaks, New York, Delacorte, 1972.

The Simultaneous Man, Bantam Books, New York, 1971.

The Foreigner, Atheneum, New York, 1961.

PEER-REVIEWED PUBLICATIONS BY MARK SCHOLZ

M. Scholz, R. Lam, R. Jennrich, et al., Prostate Cancer–Specific Survival and Clinical Progression-Free Survival in Men with Prostate Cancer Treated Intermittently with Testosterone Inactivating Pharmaceuticals. *Urology*, 70: 506, 2007.

M. Scholz, R. Lam & L. Klotz, Outcomes of Treatment versus Observation of Localized Prostate Cancer in Elderly Men, (letter). *JAMA*, 297: 1651–1652, 2007.

M. Scholz, Preventing Prostate Cancer through Diet. *Healthy Aging*, July/Aug 2006.

G. Shaw, J. Cuzick, L. Goldenberg, et al., Pragmatic Recommendation and Directions for Future Work Based on a Meta-Analysis of 1653 Patients Treated with Intermittent Hormone Therapy for Adenocarcinoma of the Prostate. *Urology*, 68(3 Supp. 5A): 2006.

M. Scholz, R. Jennrich, S. Strum, et al., Intermittent Use of Testosterone Inactivating Pharmaceuticals Using Finasteride Prolongs the Time Off Period. *Journal of Urology*, 2006.

B. Guess, M. Scholz & R. Lam, Preventing and Treating the Side Effects of

Testosterone Inactivating Pharmaceuticals in Men with Prostate Cancer. *Seminars in Preventative and Alternative Medicine*, 2006.

M. Scholz, R. Jennrich, S. Strum, et al., Long-Term Outcome in Men with Androgen Independent Prostate Cancer Treated with Ketoconazole and Hydrocortisone. *Journal of Urology*, 173: 1947, 2005.

M. Scholz, R. Lam, B. Guess & R. Blum, When Should You Start Treatment with Ketoconazole? *PAACT*, 21(#4): 2005.

M. Scholz & R. Blum, Can Diet Really Control Prostate Cancer? *PCRI Insights*, 9(1): 2006.

M. Scholz & R. Blum, Who is Really at Risk for What? *PCRI Insights*, 8(2): 2005.

M. Scholz, The Best Treatment for Prostate Cancer. *PCRI Insights*, 7(3): 2004.

B. Guess, M. Scholz, S. Strum, et al., Modified Citrus Pectin Increases the Prostate-Specific Antigen Doubling Time in Men with Prostate Cancer. *Prostate Cancer and Prostatic Diseases*, 6: 301–304, 2003.

B. Guess, R. Jennrich, H. Johnson, et al., Using Splines to Detect Changes in PSA Doubling Times. *Prostate*, 54(2): 88–94, 2003.

M. Scholz, "New Approaches to Prostate Cancer Treatment," in *Prostate Cancer Battle: It's Strictly Your Decision*, 1st Books Library, March 2002.

M. Scholz, "Early Hormone Blockade for Men Suitable for Local Therapy," in *Prostate Cancer Battle: It's Strictly Your Decision*, 1st Books Library, March 2002.

M. Scholz, R. Lam & B. Guess, "Anti-androgen Monotherapy for Prostate Cancer." *PAACT Cancer Communication Letter*, 18(2).

M. Scholz, S. Strum, F. Berrios, et al., "Low-Dose Weekly Docetaxel in Elderly Men with Prostate Cancer." *Advances in Prostate Cancer*, 5(3): 2001.

B. Guess & M. Scholz, "Re: Failure to Achieve Castrate Levels of Testosterone During Luteinizing Hormone Releasing Hormone Agonist Therapy: The Case for Monitoring Serum Testosterone and a Treatment Decision Algorithm." *Journal of Urology*, 164: 726–729, 2000.

M. Scholz & B. Strum, "PSA Nadir after Starting Hormone Blockade" (letter to the editor). *Journal of Urology*, 162: 293–306, 1999.

S. Strum, M. Scholz & J. McDermed, "Intermittent Androgen Deprivation in Prostate Cancer Patients: Factors Predictive of Prolonged Time Off Therapy." *The Oncologist* 5: 2000.

M. C. Scholz & S. B. Strum, "Recovery of Erectile Function while on Hormone Blockade Using Sildenafil (Viagra)" (letter to the editor). *Journal of Urology*, 161: 1914–1915, June 1999.

S. B. Strum, J. E. McDermed, M. C. Scholz, et al., "Anemia Associated with Androgen Deprivation (AAAD) in Prostate Cancer Patients Receiving Combination Hormone Blockade." *British Journal of Urology*, June 1997.

I. Gill, P. Gurglianone, S. M. Grunberg, et al., "High Dose Intensity of Cisplatin and Etoposide in Adenocarcinoma of Unkown Primary." *Anticancer Research*, II, 1231, 1991.

ACKNOWLEDGMENTS

RALPH H. BLUM

My portion of this book is dedicated to:

Jeanne Blum, my wife, my best friend and skilled adviser. Yourself a fine writer and formidable therapist, you kept me afloat, never shied away from hard truths, never ceased dropping honest good sense into my deaf ears, helped me clean up messes you did not make, and shared the prostate cancer journey with me from the very first day, always at my side during the darkest nights. Now I understand why so many writers use these words in their dedications: "Without you, this book could not exist." From my heart, thank you, Bones.

My abiding gratitude to:

Al Zuckerman, our agent, last of the great gentlemen editor–deal makers
Judith Gurewich, our publisher, for taking a chance on us
Corinna Barsan, our editor, for graceful and unflagging support
Yvonne Cárdenas, who made the tablecloth cover the table
Judy Blum, for endless hours of keen editing and unarguable good sense
The late Bill Blair, never at a loss to explain the hard things, sorely missed
Lawrence Bloom, brother and partner for the long haul
Larry Raithaus, MD, my 24/7 prostate cancer rabbi
Bronwyn Jones, collaborator, unfailing ally, and good companion for decades
Harvey Frost, conqueror and special mate, generous even in hard times
Judy Plowden, wise counselor and excellent friend
Bruce Lipton, PhD, and Margaret Horton, for their generosity and love
Michael Klaper, MD, my wise and generous critic and supporter
David Derris, time and again there to point out the traps and pitfalls
Steve Ravitz, black belt zen therapist and good buddy
Katherine Sky-Peck, who made time every time, however heavy her load
Rob Cowley, for sharp eyes, wit and fifty-five years of friendship
John Nolan, comrade in arms
The team at Other Press, an elegant port in an era of publishing storms
The town criers at Shreve Williams, who made sure we were visible
And to the entire staff of Prostate Oncology Specialists

If you're an amiable Refusenik, you get a lot of help. My appreciation to:

Jeff Harris, MD, Joel Friedman, MD, Duke Bahn, MD, William Coke Harrell, MD, Emily Crandall, MD, Tanya Dorff, MD, Lisa Chaiken, MD, Barry Lieberman, MD, Dick Atcheson, Tim Banse, Bill Branson, Mary Catherine Bateson, Leon Berg, Jelle Barentz, MD, Andy Bowers, Bill Chastain, Richard Cohen, Carolyn Conger, Randolph d'Amore, Helen Divov, Phil Slater, Steve Stein, Ken Wolkoff, MD, Father Henry Joe Johnson, Jerry Parr, Lloyd Costello, MD, Mary Cossette, Susan Adams Kennedy, Jerome Goldstein, Burton Greene, Viktor Gurewich, MD, Dene Lusby, Heather Paul, David Hiemens, Bill Hushion, John "Rowdy" Yeats, Bob Jacobs, Melissa Licker, Alexei Kirilloff, Spencer Feldman, Bob Chartoff, John Alexander, Jeremy Tarcher, Liz Rich, Alan Slifka, Sir Christopher Mallaby, Shelley St. John, John Kurhanowicz, PhD, Richard Lamb, MD, Starling Lawrence, Ben Levi, Andrew Beath, Kenny Loggins, Charlie Lustman, Monique Fey, Alec Cast, Aaron Kipnis, Angel Thompson, Stan Madson, Robert Wilkinson, Dorian and Jeffrey Bergen, Paul Brenner, MD, Beth Gagnon, Duncan Denny, Akani Fletcher, Kari Andrikopolis, Melody Mendenhall, Ray Montella, Leslie "Nosher" Neale, Suzanne Taylor, Ted Ravinett, Jerry Moss, Judith Praeger, Thorsten Orlikowsky, MD, Ruth Marlin, MD, Linda Lou Prestyly, Steve Ravitz, Wally Reid, Loren White, Susan Weed, Furuku Takaheshi, MD, Toni Wilbanks, Sebastian Rice-Edwards, Sally Richardson, Stephan Schwartz, Phil Thompson, Bill Whitson, Judy Skutch Whitson, David Young, Tracy Tucker and the much missed Brad Guest, James Coburn, Judd Huss, John Michell, Pierre Cossette, Harry Pinchon, and Robert Ott.

Finally my very special thanks to:

The prostate cancer guys: a veritable task force of outstanding men I have had the privilege of learning from and talking story with over the past twenty years; men who faced the unknown with courage, honesty, intelligence and good humor. You have opened our eyes to a new vision of prostate cancer as manageable, liable to holding in check and survivable no matter what the odds. Not only is this book written for you, it is made possible by you. Without my cancer, I'd have missed out on knowing some great people. Let our motto be: "*Die with it, not from it.*"

And wherever memory's net has failed, and a name has slipped out, forgive me. In the night, when sleep fans the embers of gratitude, I will remember you and bless you.

MARK SCHOLZ

My heartfelt appreciation to Juliet, my dear wife, who endured my absence and still prayed for the success of the project. To Dennis, my very special mother, who has the gift to see the potential in others and find a way to nurture it. To Ralph, my coauthor, whose conviction, talent, professionalism and expertise made the book happen. To Richard Lam, MD, my partner, Jill Peck and Melody Mendenhall, my nurses, to Kaili Shewmaker, my office manager, and to Father Joe Johnson and Barry Clark, who kindly read portions of the book and rendered invaluable advice. To John Sarian, Rol Christian and Will Rogers, best buddies who love me enough to "tell it like it is." To the rest of my great family for their loving prayers and support. Also to Adriane Friedman, my great teacher at Occidental College, who gave me my first practical introduction to writing. And lastly, my grateful appreciation for Judith Gurewich, our publisher, and Corinna Barsan and Yvonne Cárdenas, our editors, and the rest of the team at Other Press who made this whole venture possible.

INDEX

Abiraterone, 223
Acosta, Judith, LCSW, 178
active surveillance, 24, 128, 131, 136
    after Combidex MRI, 144
    benefits of, 169, 221
    as best treatment for Low-Risk cancer,
        69, 78, 145–146, 228
    resistance to, 8–9, 60, 63–64, 69, 79
    results of, 66–68
    safety of, 68, 86, 228
Actonel, to control side effects of lack of
    testosterone, 149
acupuncture, 24–25
Adler, Robert, PhD, 197
Advanced Magnetics, Combidex by,
    137, 156–163
age, 134, 213–214
    active surveillance and, 66–67
    influence on libido, 89, 147
    prostate enlarging with, 82, 84
    risks of surgery and, 19, 22, 43
aggressiveness, of prostate cancer. See
    also High-Risk cancer
    evaluating, 7n, 82–84, 86, 121
    influences on, 171, 175–176,
        189–190
alternative medicine, 24–26, 36. See
    also specific modalities
American Cancer Society, 26–27, 50
Anatomy of an Illness (Cousins), 206
Anderson, Greg, 201–203, 219
androgen deprivation therapy. See hor-
    mone blockade
anesthesia, general, 116, 179
angiogenesis (blood flow to tumor), ultra-
    sound imaging of, 35, 58, 131, 221
animal products, in diet, 173–176,
    189–191, 194

antibiotics, 20, 49, 85
antidepressants, 149
antioxidants, 171, 191–192, 206
APeX Solution, 34–36, 225
Arigo, José, 32
arthritis, from lack of testosterone, 149
attitude. See emotions
Aubin, Sylvie, PhD, 53
auricular therapy, 24–25
Avodart, 35, 86, 99, 102

Bach, Peter, MD, 21n
Bahn, Duke, MD, 57
    biopsy by, 103–104
    cryosurgery by, 104, 132
    monitoring tumors with ultrasound,
        35, 58, 129, 136
    urologist and, 105–108
Barentsz, Jelle, MD, 137, 142
Be Careful What You Pray For... You
    Just Might Get It (Dossey), 179
Beating Cancer with Nutrition (Quil-
    lin), 201
beliefs, influence of, 180, 184–186,
    202–203, 207, 219–220
benign prostatic hyperplasia (BPH), 79,
    82, 84, 86, 153
Benson, Herbert, MD, 181
The Biology of Belief (Lipton), 56
biopsies
    active surveillance and, 68
    avoiding unnecessary, 19, 58, 81–82,
        85–86, 127, 130–131, 221
    color Doppler ultrasound directed,
        130, 134, 136
    crush artifacts in, 2, 6–7
    in diagnosis, 6, 11, 41